Baby Boys

Baby boys

❤ An Owner's Manual ❤

THERESA FOY DIGERONIMO, M.ED.

Foreword by Stephen E. Muething, M.D.

A Perigee Book

THE BERKLEY PUBLISHING GROUP
Published by the Penguin Group
Penguin Group (USA) Inc.
375 Hudson Street, New York, New York 10014, USA
Penguin Group (Canada), 90 Eglinton Avenue East, Suite 700, Toronto, Ontario M4P 2Y3, Canada
(a division of Pearson Penguin Canada Inc.)
Penguin Books Ltd., 80 Strand, London WC2R 0RL, England
Penguin Group Ireland, 25 St. Stephen's Green, Dublin 2, Ireland (a division of Penguin Books Ltd.)
Penguin Group (Australia), 250 Camberwell Road, Camberwell, Victoria 3124, Australia
(a division of Pearson Australia Group Pty. Ltd.)
Penguin Books India Pvt. Ltd., 11 Community Centre, Panchsheel Park, New Delhi—110 017, India
Penguin Group (NZ), Cnr. Airborne and Rosedale Roads, Albany, Auckland 1310, New Zealand
(a division of Pearson New Zealand Ltd.)
Penguin Books (South Africa) (Pty.) Ltd., 24 Sturdee Avenue, Rosebank, Johannesburg 2196,
South Africa

Penguin Books Ltd., Registered Offices: 80 Strand, London WC2R 0RL, England

Copyright © 2005 by Literary Productions
Text design by Tiffany Estreicher
Cover art and design by Liz Sheehan

PRINTING HISTORY
Perigee trade paperback edition / December 2005

PERIGEE is a registered trademark of Penguin Group (USA) Inc.
The "P" design is a trademark belonging to Penguin Group (USA) Inc.

Library of Congress Cataloging-in-Publication Data

DiGeronimo, Theresa Foy.
    Baby boys : a complete guide to your son's first 18 months / by Theresa Foy
DeGeronimo ; foreword by Stephen E. Meuthing.
       p.   cm.
    "Developed by Literary Productions."
    "A Perigee Book."
    Includes bibliographical references.
    ISBN 0-399-53209-9
    1. Infant boys—Health and hygiene.   2. Infant boys—Care.   I. Title.

RJ61.D56   2005
649'.132—dc22

                                                      2005043254

PRINTED IN THE UNITED STATES OF AMERICA

10   9   8   7   6   5   4   3   2   1

To my sons, Matt and Joe.
Your marvelous adventures and antics
have given life to this book—and to me.

Contents

One

It's a Boy! Now What?

Two

Bright Beginnings:
Your Boy from Birth Through Three Months

Three
Settling In:
Your Boy from Four to Seven Months

Four
Movers and Shakers:
Your Boy from Eight to Eleven Months

Five

A Toddler in the House:
Your Boy from Twelve to Eighteen Months . . . and Beyond

Physical Growth   228
Get Up and Go 228

Emotional Development   229
For Security Sake 230 / Big Boys Do Cry 230

Cognitive Development   231
Boys and Their Legos 232 / The Strong Silent Type 233 / Learning to Pretend 236

Social Development   239
Making Friends 239 / Imaginary Friends 242

Acting Like a Boy   243
Where Do They Get These Ideas? 244 / What Do They Learn? 249 / What's a Parent to Do? 251

Becoming a Little Man   251

Foreword

When my first son, Ted, was born, I remember feeling incredible pride. I had just finished medical school and was completing my pediatric residency at the time. My wife, Meg, and I already had two daughters, so the idea of being a parent was nothing new. But even with all of our previous experiences, not to mention my background in pediatrics, I was still taken by how different Ted was from my girls.

Having come from a family of seven boys, and being male myself, I figured raising a son would be a piece of cake. That wasn't quite the case. For instance, while my girls preferred being caressed and soothed, Ted loved being tossed around. And though our girls were rather quiet as babies, Ted was into everything. He even wanted to play with different kinds of toys than the girls did and was far more independent. In many respects, having a baby boy was like starting the parenting process all over again, even though our oldest daughter was already five.

Without a doubt, it would have been great to have a copy of *Baby Boys* to help get me through these times. There were so many things my wife and I didn't know and understand about our son, his needs, and his behaviors. While my observations were mostly anecdotal back then, after twelve years in private practice and now as associate director of clinical services at Cincinnati Children's Hospital Medical Center, I can assure you from a medical perspective that there are some big differences between boys and girls in everything from their health to the way they act.

Right from the start, boys are more likely to be born premature. They are more susceptible to having attention deficit disorder, have more aggressive personalities, can be hot-tempered, are more prone to accidents, have bigger and more varied appetites, are more competitive, and enter puberty a couple of years later than girls. These differences even extend to such areas as toilet training. Boys are far less open to having people in the room with them while learning to use the potty. Instead, they like their privacy. The list goes on and on, but I think you get the idea. And these differences will only increase as your son grows older.

I always tell parents that raising a child is the most important job they'll ever have. Since we're all poorly prepared for this awesome responsibility, it would be nice if we could have a specific owner's manual to guide us through the parenting process for our baby. The book you are holding in your hands goes a long way toward fitting this bill in a way that's quite unique from anything else out there today.

In the pages that follow, Theresa Foy DiGeronimo—a parenting expert in her own right—will lead you through what you need to know as you raise your wonderful boy from birth through the early toddler years. In addition to presenting you with the latest research and medical findings, Theresa will share with you her own personal experiences in raising her two boys. (She also has a daughter, so she's witnessed the differences firsthand.)

Knowing the basics will go a long way toward making you the best parent you can be. This book will show you how to care for your boy, how to feed him, and how to keep him safe. It will also help you to better understand your son's own individuality, including the nuances of his body and personality and great ways to keep him happy. By understanding your son's unique traits—and how boys differ from girls—you'll have a solid head start in doing the greatest job of all.

Now, before you get started on this journey, let me leave you with a bit of parting advice. First, whether you're still expecting or have already welcomed your baby boy to the world, don't be surprised if you're a little scared. It's perfectly normal to feel like you may be in over your head, while fearing you'll do something wrong. Just about every new parent feels this way. I sure did.

The important thing is for you to take care of your son the best way you know how, and also to take good care of your partner. You're in this together and need each other now more than ever. Slow down your lives and take everything day by day. You're going to be exhausted, especially in your son's first few months. Then, as time goes by, you'll begin to realize that you're getting the hang of this parenting thing. You'll be more at ease, and you'll sleep better at night.

If you already have a daughter, and this is your first boy, I'll add this bit of advice: Hang on! It's going to be a much different ride. You will have to change your parenting style to adjust to your son's unique needs. Fortunately, a lot of the basics in the early years are the same, so it won't be quite as scary as it was the first time around. But it will be different, and this book will help you to deal with that.

The good news is that early successes in parenting build on each other. As a result, if you are able to understand, accept, and deal with these smaller differences now, you are bound to be better prepared to handle the big stuff that's sure to come as your son grows older. After all, the teenage years will be here before you know it!

So get ready for what's bound to be a wonderful journey as you raise your new son. Remember, it's okay to make mistakes, and the more you know and understand about your boy going in, the better you'll be able to cope with the many wonderful adventures you are about to encounter.

Stephen E. Muething, M.D.
Associate director of clinical services,
Cincinnati Children's Hospital Medical Center
Assistant professor, Pediatrics, University of Cincinnati

Introduction

I have raised two boys through the ups and downs of babyhood and know for sure that there's nothing like having a son! He is a full-speed-ahead bundle of energy with muddied hands, messy pockets, and sticky kisses. He is infuriating and at the same time lovable, and a true blessing at the end of every day. I've also found that there is so much to learn about little boys and so little time to do it before they're all grown up.

Baby Boys: An Owner's Manual is a road map for your bundle of joy's earliest years, from setting up the nursery to selecting just the right foods. As both a mother and the author of numerous parenting books on a variety of topics, I'll open the doors to giving you a better understanding of just how and why boys are so different from girls, including the latest research into this topic from the many recognized experts I have turned to for advice and guidance.

Baby Boys brings you into the world of snips and snails and puppy dog tails, while examining the physical, cognitive, and emotional makeup of boys to help you to better understand your newly formed XY chromosome miracle. It gives you information, tips, and advice about pressing parenting issues and concerns—while always keeping an eye on the world from your little boy's point of view.

While the book is divided by age range, you may find it interesting to read the book from start to finish so you get a complete picture of all the factors that influence the development of a male from birth through around eighteen months. Then, refer to each section over and over again as your son moves through these first five critical stages of childhood. You'll come away not only with better parenting skills, but also with answers to such questions as "Why does he always act that way?" and "Is it really normal for boys to do that?"

Without a doubt, by the time you're through, you'll have a much better understanding of what boys are made of, along with the knowledge of what you can do to prepare for this new lifelong adventure.

One

It's A Boy! Now What?

It's a boy—congratulations! Through the marvels of modern medicine, you may know you're going to have a baby boy before you've even given birth. How wonderful to know your son, to feel his high kicks, and to call him by name before the two of you have formally met. Or, you may be reading this book after you've already held your son, kissed his forehead, and wondered in a panic: *Now what!?* Either way, this book will get you going in the right direction.

In this chapter, we'll explore some of the basics you need to prepare, even before bringing your son home from the hospital. In a moment, we'll talk about selecting a doctor and getting your baby boy's room set up. But first we'll discuss one of the most basic decisions you'll have to make (and also one of the most enjoyable): finding the right name for your bundle of joy.

Naming Your Son

I've given my boys very conventional names: Matthew and Joseph. But there's obviously no law limiting what you can call your son. Comedian and civil rights leader, Dick Gregory, gave his twins the middle names of Inte and Gration. George Foreman named all four of his sons George. And Michael Jackson named his two boys Prince Michael I and Prince Michael II.

Choosing just the right name can be a tough task, but be glad you have the choice. Your task of choosing among thousands of possible names for your son is a relatively new dilemma—the practice is only about three hundred years old in the Western European world. Before that time, there was a rather strict code that named the firstborn son after the father's father, the second son after the mother's father, the third son after the father himself, and later sons after the baby's uncles. Everyone was named after a family member. This did not allow for much change or variety from generation to generation.

So, if you're naming your son after his father or grandfather (as I did), you're on solid historical ground and in good company. Although it's no longer the rule, American boys today are still far more likely to be named after a relative than are females (although this tradition is slowly changing) and those generational names are often common names like Joseph, Michael, Matthew, and

Robert. These names wear well in our society as boys age into adulthood.

Dr. Cleveland Kent Evans of the American Name Society believes that common, traditional names are given to males more often than to females because our society does not use male names to differentiate the bearer. Males are expected to go out and "make a name" for themselves. They will be judged not on the superficial name, but rather on their accomplishments. Girls, on the other hand, are frequently given unique or fanciful names to distinguish them from other girls because traditionally they were not expected to distinguish themselves by the lives they lived.

However, this long-standing tradition of passing on family names generation after generation is changing rapidly. Many families are

A POPULARITY CONTEST

According to a recent report by the Social Security Administration, the most popular male names as this book went to press were:

1. Jacob
2. Michael
3. Joshua
4. Matthew
5. Ethan
6. Andrew
7. Daniel
8. William
9. Joseph
10. Christopher

You can find more information from the Social Security Administration about popular baby names at:

http://www.ssa.gov/OACT/babynames.

now looking outside the family tree for male names. Dr. Evans notes that during the 1990s, less than half of all newborn boys were given one of the top fifty historically most popular names.

With more freedom to choose male names outside the immediate family, some parents decide to honor their roots by choosing an ethnic or religious name. Muhammad Ali chose to do this, for example, by naming his children Maryum, Muhammed Jr., Rasheeda, Jamila, Miya, Khalilah, Hana, Laila, and Asaad. Dr. Evans has noticed that first-generation immigrants will often give their children American-sounding names to help them fit in with the society. But by the third generation some parents feel pride in their ancestry and make that feeling known by giving their children ethnic or religious names. This is nothing new. Back at the turn of the nineteenth century, when Irish immigrants were brutally persecuted, there was not a Kevin, Patrick, or Sean to be found. But two generations later, many Irish lads proudly wore those names.

QUICK CHECKLIST FOR CHOOSING YOUR SON'S NAME

As you're tossing around possible names for your son, keep these tips in mind to help you make a decision you and your child can live with for many years to come:

- ☐ **Say it out loud.** Does the first name and your last name flow nicely and sound good together? Do they bang into each other and trip up the tongue? Or do they make you laugh (think Newton Hooton)?

GIVE ME A BOY!

Your baby boy gives you something that most American parents want—a son! A Gallup Organization poll has asked adults every few years since 1941 what they would choose if they could only have a son or a daughter. The findings have consistently favored boys. The most recent survey of 1,003 adults in 2003 found:

- Among men, 45 percent preferred a boy, and 19 percent a girl. Twenty-nine percent had no preference.

- Among women, 36 percent wanted a girl, and 32 percent a boy. Twenty-six percent had no preference.

The percentages do not add up to 100 percent because some respondents gave no opinion.

☐ **Does the name you're thinking of have a nickname?** If you don't like the nickname, stay away from the proper name. Once kids reach school, you may lose control of what the other children call your son. Benjamin can become Benji whether you like it or not.

☐ **Check out the initials.** I planned to name my firstborn Matthew Adam, but then realized his initials would be M.A.D. and quickly changed my mind.

☐ **Consider gender identification.** There are several names and nicknames that can be male or female, such as Lynn, Leslie,

Sam, or Chris. If you choose such a name, your child will be plagued with name problems for the rest of his life. My neighbor's daughter arrived for her first day of college to find that her roommate Chris was male, requiring a quick reshuffling of room assignments, and much embarrassment for poor Chris.

Selecting Your Son's Doctor

The doctor who looks in on your son immediately after his birth may not be the one you want to stick with in the long run. Because your son's doctor will care for his medical needs from birth to approximately age eighteen, you should choose this long-term relationship carefully.

OPTIONS TO CONSIDER

When choosing your son's physician, here are some things to think about:

Pediatrician or Family Practitioner: A pediatrician is a physician who specializes in the development, care, and diseases of children. A family practitioner is a physician who has training in many areas of medicine and can be the primary care provider for all members of your family. Both are qualified to care for your baby. When making the choice, you have to decide if you would like your son in the care of someone who has specialized training with babies and children, or if you'd like someone who knows and cares for you, too. If your son is healthy with no special needs, choose the doctor you are most comfortable with. But if your son has any medical problems that require careful monitoring, many families find it best to select a pediatrician with specialized training in the particular childhood illness and its treatment.

Insurance Considerations: If you have insurance, you may want to narrow your search by choosing a doctor who participates in your health-care plan. Your provider may have given you a booklet or a website listing all participating doctors in your area. You can also call member services and ask for help in locating doctors near you.

Of course you can go out of network to a doctor who is not a participating physician, but it will cost you. Unlike most healthy adults who may see a doctor once or twice a year, routine childhood checkups and illnesses are quite frequent and the bills can pile up quickly. Before you sign up with an out-of-network physician, find out exactly how much the cost will be for each checkup, emergency care, and for hospital care. Then make your decision.

Location: It's a good idea to stick close to home. Children commonly need quick emergency treatment for high fevers, deep cuts, and the like. Long trips to a distant physician will soon wear you out.

Male or Female: Your infant son will not care about the gender of his doctor. But as he grows, this can become an issue. I found that my baby boys were more comfortable with a female when they were sick or in pain, and therefore were calmer with their female physician. But as they grew into adolescence and puberty, they preferred a male doctor. Perhaps the best of all worlds is found in a group practice that would allow you to choose a female doctor while your son is young and a male doctor later if that would make him feel more at ease.

GET A RECOMMENDATION

As you narrow down your preferences be sure to ask around for recommendations. A physician may look impressive on paper based on his or her education and position in the medical community, but only those families who rely on a doctor for medical care really know how he or she handles worried parents and sick children.

You might first ask your obstetrician. (Ask who he or she uses for his or her own kids!) Also, talk to friends and family members who have already chosen a doctor for their children. Ask questions such as:

- Does your doctor welcome questions?

- Does he take time to discuss problems and listen to your concerns?

- Is the office staff pleasant and helpful?

- How long do you wait in the waiting room? (This becomes a very important consideration when your child is sick and ill-tempered.)

- Does the waiting room have a separate area for sick children?

- How quickly does she return your calls?

- Does your child like the doctor?

Based on all this information, make a list of the top few physicians you might choose and go out and meet them.

INTERVIEWING POTENTIAL DOCTORS

Time is tight at a bustling doctor's office, so it's never a good idea to drop in for a "surprise" interview. But if you plan ahead, most physicians will agree to talk with you about their practice. (Many physicians offer half-hour consultations for a nominal charge.) Call each doctor's office and ask if you can set up a potential-patient interview. Some doctors will have time only for a phone conversation, while others will invite you to the office. (If you have to settle for a phone call, be sure to visit the office to look around the waiting area before making your final decision. There's a lot you can learn from the state of cleanliness, organization, and crowding of the office that you can't get over the phone.) The kind of response you get for your request for an interview will perhaps tell you all you need to know about a physician who is too busy, too important, or too disinterested to meet with a new parent.

Use your interview time to ask questions about the practical aspects of the doctor's practice as well as his or her beliefs and philosophy. For example, you might ask:

- What are the office hours? Are you available on weekends? How are emergencies on holidays or middle-of-the-night calls handled?

- If this is a group practice, will my child see the same doctor at each checkup?

- At which hospital do you have full staff privileges?

- Do sick children use the same waiting room as healthy kids for routine checkups?

- Who is your covering doctor when you're not available?

- What is your payment and billing policy?

- What is your advice about how to handle a crying baby?

SELECTING A PEDIATRICIAN

You can get the names of doctors who are certified by the American Board of Pediatrics from:

- Your local medical society

- A hospital referral service

- The American Academy of Pediatrics (AAP). Send a self-addressed, stamped envelope to: Pediatric Referral Department, AAP, PO Box 927, Elk Grove Village, IL 60009. Be sure to mention which region of the country you're interested in.

- If I have trouble breast-feeding, will I be able to call you for help?

The office staff might be able to answer some of the practical questions before your interview, leaving you more time to ask the doctor about his feelings and opinions on child-care matters that are most important to you. The person you choose will care for your child into his teen years, so be sure it is someone you like and trust.

Getting Ready for Your Baby Boy

The list of baby things you'll want to buy before your baby boy arrives is, of course, endless, but here are a few items that experienced parents say they were glad to have in the house before delivery day.

BABY CLOTHES

Little boy clothes are so cute! We all fall in love with the tiny three-piece suits (bow tie and all), and I clearly remember the jogging outfits with miniature sneakers that I just *had* to have for my sons. But although it is tempting to buy a carload of these adorable outfits, I learned the hard way that boys barely have a chance to go out on the town before they outgrow their infant clothing. It's usually best to leave the buying of fancy duds to relatives and friends, and focus your purchasing power on a practical day-to-day wardrobe that includes the following:

- ☐ At least six stretchy, snap-up-the-front, one-piece pajamas with feet. These are the most useful fashion wear for newborns. They live in them!

- ☐ At least a half-dozen front-snapping tee shirts or one-piece snap-crotch tees.

- ☐ Another half-dozen pairs of socks or booties. (Booties that tie around the ankle will stay on longer than socks.)

- ☐ A hat. Whether the forecast calls for a wool hat or a sun hat, you'll want to keep your baby's head covered.

- ☐ A snowsuit, if you live in a cold region.

DIAPERS

You wouldn't be the first parent to bring home a new baby and realize an hour later that babies need diapers. Get them now. If you are using disposable diapers, look for the newborn size with a cutout around the navel. However, don't buy too many because your baby will quickly outgrow them. They are good for about three weeks, at the most, while your baby's cord stump is drying out.

If you're using cloth diapers, purchase about six dozen in size large (they can be folded to fit your baby at each stage of growth). You might also consider buying diaper liners, which absorb small amounts of urine and are easily changed without adding another full diaper to the laundry load. You'll also need six diaper wraps, or plastic pants, and six pairs of diaper pins.

In addition to diapers, you'll need diapering supplies. Buy a tube of ointment to prevent diaper rash, but make it a small one. You may have to try a brand or two until you find one that works best on your son. Many doctors say it's best to stay away from commercial baby wipes when changing a newborn; they have been known to cause harsh reactions on a baby's soft bottom. Stick to sterile cotton balls dipped in warm water for cleanups.

HEALTH AND GROOMING AIDS

There are a few items you might want to have on hand when your baby arrives. The following will take care of any minor health problems in the first few weeks and also keep your baby well groomed:

☐ **Cool-mist humidifier:** Dry air is tough on little nostrils. A cool-mist humidifier will help your baby breathe more easily.

☐ **Bulb syringe:** Even with a humidifier in the room, it's likely that your baby will still get the occasional stuffy nose. Until he learns to blow his nose like the rest of us, the bulb syringe is the best way to remove mucus from a congested nose.

☐ **Rectal thermometer:** It will be a while before you can use the family oral thermometer to check your son's temperature. The rectal type is a must—either mercury or digital. And pick up some petroleum jelly to coat the thermometer before use for easy insertion.

☐ **Rounded-tipped scissor or baby nail clipper:** You'll be amazed how quickly little baby finger- and toenails grow! The finger-

IT'S ALL IN THE BRAIN

Before a child is even born there are noticeable differences between the male and female brain. At six weeks, the male brain gets a large dose of male hormone that changes the brain permanently and determines sexual identity. A boy's brain is 10 percent larger in mass than a girl's, but the corpus callosum (which connects the two hemispheres of the brain and helps coordinate the activities of the left and right hemisphere) is smaller. The male brain also produces less serotonin—a quieting agent—which may explain why boys seem to be more active in the womb.

nails especially must be kept very short so your baby won't scratch the delicate skin on his face.

☐ **Comb and/or hairbrush:** Adult and big-kid combs and brushes can scratch a newborn's scalp. Get one designed specifically for newborns with soft brush bristles and rounded comb teeth.

BABY BATHTUB

Some folks say that you can bathe an infant in any plastic tub, in the sink, or in the bathtub with a towel under him to prevent slipping. While this is true, bathing a young son is a slippery business. That's why a baby bathtub specially molded for infants can be a big help, especially if you're not practiced in the art of baby handling.

The tub should be made of plastic heavy enough not to bend under the weight of a full load of water. It should have a plug for draining the water, a slip-resistant bottom, and be shaped to hold the baby in a semi-upright position on a slip-resistant surface. For a longer period of usefulness, get a tub designed for both infants and toddlers. Indentations to hold washcloths, soap, and a cup (for rinsing) are nice features.

Whatever you choose, you won't use the tub and submerge the baby's belly into the water until he is a couple of weeks old and the umbilical cord stump has healed. Until then, you'll just use a washcloth or sponge for daily cleaning. (For more on bathing your infant, see chapter 2.)

BABY MONITOR

An audio baby monitor lets you eavesdrop on your baby when he is out of sight. It consists of a transmitter that is placed in the baby's room and a portable receiver that can be put in another room or carried around to hear the baby's cries, sighs, and breath-

MONITOR WARNING

Baby monitor transmissions can be picked up on cell phones as well as on neighbors' baby monitor receivers. So be careful what you say in the baby's room—many a parent has had an embarrassingly frank conversation before remembering the transmitter was on.

ing. Volume is adjustable and some have visual cues, such as red lights that flash when a sound registers.

You might also think about going high-tech with a video monitor. These are available at most baby supply stores and are easy to install and use. They consist of a video camera that you can train on your sleeping baby, and a small (4 × 5") television monitor that you can keep nearby whereever you are in the house.

These monitors, whether audio or video, can be reassuring devices. They're especially comforting if you're a sound sleeper and your baby sleeps in another room, or if you have a large house and want to be alerted when your baby wakes from his nap.

Setting Up Your Baby Boy's Room

As my little family grew, we moved from an apartment to a small house to a larger house. In each home I set up another nursery! It was always so much fun imagining a new infant in the room and selecting just the right color scheme, bedding, changing table, and toys.

Since I'm no expert on decorating a baby boy's nursery, I contacted Laurie Smith, the much-loved designer on TLC's *Trading Spaces*. Laurie created a nursery for her son, Gibson Witherspoon (named after his great-grandfather), which was featured in a special baby edition of *Parents* magazine.

"I think many young parents get overwhelmed thinking that they must know the sex of the baby before it's born in order to have the nursery completely decorated when the baby arrives," says Laurie with a laugh. "Call me resourceful, but I just think it's fun to have a basic, gender-neutral room to decorate with boyish or girlish elements—without painting the whole room blue or pink."

So, while Laurie was pregnant, she created a nursery that would work for either a girl or a boy since she wanted to be surprised on the delivery day, and also because it seemed more practical to her. "I wanted to use bedding, fabrics, and wall color that could be used again for a boy or a girl because I don't want to have to reinvest in a whole new nursery when baby number two comes along. This allowed me to invest in a higher-quality crib and bedding and draperies because I knew they would be used for several years with two children, and that made the extra expense worthwhile."

Laurie says it was fun to make a bright, fun room, knowing she could embellish with things like a throw rug or crib mobile to be more boyish or more girlish when the time came. "But the key," she says, "was to use vibrant, bright colors that would stimulate the baby and be a catalyst for thought and imagination."

As a designer, Laurie always tells parents to start a space with something that inspires them and go from there. "For my baby's nursery," she confides, "I found a bedding fabric that I thought was precious and that guided all my color selections. The fabric has yellow, green, and tints of red in it. These are wonderfully gender-neutral colors with nice depth that give the room its foundation. That led me to a drapery of yellow with tiny veins of red and vivid yellow-green. I used the same green to paint the walls and then bought white furniture. The room has hardwood floors, and after Gibson was born and I knew I was decorating for a boy, I bought this 'boyish' throw rug for the area by the crib that has farm animals and a barn on it. And I bought a crib mobile with little ducks."

Although Laurie certainly spent time mapping out the look of Gibson's room, she says she has seen too many parents make the mistake of getting caught up in the look of the nursery without giving enough time and attention to its function. "A young mother came to me upset because her beautiful window treatments didn't block out the sunlight and her baby wouldn't go down for a nap. The aesthetics of the room were wonderful, but sometimes parents forget that the baby will actually live there and will need the room to be functional as well. It can be fun and fanciful (to please the parents) and still be a good place for a baby to sleep and play."

Laurie was pleased that she designed function into Gibson's room after learning that baby boys are into everything and move a mile a minute. "I'm so glad," she says with obvious relief, "that he has a comfortable area where he can turn his back on me and enjoy his space. There's absolutely nothing in there that can hurt him. So it's the one place in the house where he can move around without being told 'No!' I also designated a wonderful area in the room that has low, accessible shelves for Gibson's books and toys. This is a place where he can access things and explore on his own without waiting for me to get things down for him. I think it's important for babies to have a room that they can explore safely on their own."

So there you have it—straight from a designer's mouth. Create a safe, playful environment for your son. And go for vibrant, gender-neutral colors, adding accessories that say "A baby boy lives here."

Safety First

As you're choosing the furniture for your baby's nursery, here are few tips to help you decorate, keeping style and safety in mind.

BABY BED

Your son's first bed is an important purchase. It is the one place he will spend most of his time until he's up on his feet and running, so it's important to make sure it is a safe place—whether bassinet, cradle, or crib.

Bassinet or Cradle: Who can resist the beauty of a lacy bassinet or the polished wood of an infant cradle? Either one is an ideal addition to any nursery. The bassinet for my first son was covered entirely with white lace and had the traditional hooded design. I loved it and was very disappointed when after only three weeks, he grew too long for its diminutive size and was kicking so hard at the sides I worried about its stability. This was probably my first lesson in how quickly our babies grow.

The U.S. Consumer Product Safety Commission (CPSC) warns that the most frequent injury associated with bassinets and cradles involves children falling either when the bottom of the bassinet or cradle breaks, or when it tips over or collapses. Suffocation has also been reported in products that are not structurally sound, or when pillows or folded quilts were under the baby.

If you buy a bassinet or cradle, keep these CPSC tips in mind:

☐ Look for one with a sturdy bottom and a wide, stable base.

☐ Follow the manufacturer's guidelines on the appropriate weight and size of baby who can safely use the bassinet or cradle.

☐ Check to make sure that spaces between spindles are no larger than 2⅜ inches.

☐ Check screws and bolts periodically to ensure they are tight.

☐ If the product has legs that fold for storage, make sure that effective locks are provided to ensure the legs don't accidentally fold while in use.

☐ Mattresses and padding should fit snugly and be firm and smooth. *Never use pillows for padding*.

☐ Decorative bows and ribbons should be trimmed short and stitched securely to prevent strangulation.

☐ Swinging cradles should have a way to prevent them from swinging once a baby is asleep.

Baby Crib: After some dusty digging, I found my old baby crib in my parents' basement. I actually remembered being in this crib (or maybe I remembered the many pictures I've seen of me standing at its rails). It was an adorable, soft cream color with stenciled pale green teddy bears on the headboard. But after setting it up and standing back to admire it, I got a sinking feeling that what passed for "state-of-the-art" years ago wouldn't be safe or sturdy enough for my son.

The best investment you can make for your baby is a crib that

CRIBS: SAFETY CHECKLIST

☐ Slats are spaced no more than 2⅜ inches (60 mm) apart.

☐ No slats are missing, loose, or cracked.

☐ Mattress fits snugly—no more than two fingers' width between edge of mattress and cribside.

☐ Mattress support is securely attached to the headboard and footboard.

☐ Corner posts are no higher than 1/16 of an inch (1½ mm).

☐ No cutouts in top edge of headboard and footboard.

☐ Drop-side latches cannot be easily released by your baby.

☐ Drop-side latches securely hold side in raised position.

☐ All screws, bolts and other hardware are present and tight.

meets all of CPSC's safety standards. This is important because according to the CPSC, cribs account for more deaths of infants than any other nursery item—and each year, thousands of infants are injured seriously enough in cribs to require treatment in hospital emergency rooms.

CHANGING TABLE

In the first year or so, you'll spend a lot of time changing your son's diapers. Therefore, a solid and safe changing table is a good investment—and also the best way to prevent the backaches you'd get from bending over to change your son's diapers while he's lying on your bed or on the floor.

The changing table you choose should have room for storing changing supplies so you never have to leave your baby unattended to grab a diaper or ointment. It must also have a safety strap that is easy to use. The CPSC says that over 1,300 infants a year are injured in changing-table-related accidents. Most of these injuries occur when babies fall from the changing table to the floor. So look for one with a good strap, and then be sure to use it. (And remember: Just because you are using the safety straps doesn't mean that you can leave your child unattended.)

For Boys on the Go

It won't be long before you and your son are out and about. There are a few pieces of equipment you might want to have in the house before your baby boy arrives to make travel safe and easy. These include a diaper bag, front carrier, car seat, carrier seat, and stroller.

DIAPER BAG

Every time you leave home with your baby, your diaper bag will go with you, so look for one that will hold up for the long haul. It should be washable and contain an insulated compartment for keeping bottles warm or cool. It should have multiple compartments for organizing the many baby items you'll need to find quickly (pacifier, baby wipes, rattle, bottles, diapers, ointment, burp cloth, and on and on). You should consider buying the bag in a design and color (other than pastel baby prints) that the baby's dad will also feel comfortable carrying.

FRONT CARRIER

You'll quickly find that newborn babies love to be held close to your heart. You'll also soon discover that doing this all day long makes it difficult to do anything else! That's why so many new parents love their baby carriers. Front carriers are best for newborns because they provide extra head support. You'll notice that front carriers come in many different designs and shapes: Some look like a sling, which hold the baby in a prone position; others are more sacklike and hold the baby upright against your chest. Either way, your son will be kept warm, cozy, and near your heart. As your baby grows and gains weight, you'll probably want to switch to a back carrier, which puts less strain on your own back and gives your son more opportunity to look around.

CAR SEAT

By law, all children under age five must be strapped into a car seat when riding in a car. This is so important that most hospitals will not release a baby until they are assured the parent has a car seat in the vehicle that will be taking the baby home. That's why you should make this purchase before delivery.

Because your baby will use a car seat for several years, it's worth your time to do some comparison shopping. Here are some basics to help you make the right choice. Car seats are made in two basic styles:

Infant seat: This is designed for children under twenty pounds and faces the back of the car.

Infant-toddler seat: This can be used by both infants and older children up to forty pounds. It faces the back for infant use, and is turned around to face front when the baby reaches twenty pounds.

When you are comparing car seats, look for:

- **Price.** They run from around $50 to $200. Somewhere in the middle is probably the best buy.

- **Easy installation.** If you can't install the seat correctly every time you put it in the car, it won't protect your baby properly. Make sure you feel comfortable with the installation process before you buy.

- **Seat belt adjustments.** Check out how the seat belt from the car gets attached to the car seat. Some are easy; some require an engineering degree.

- **Washability.** If this is your first baby, you have no idea how messy the car seat can become. All kinds of dirt, food, drink, and vomited substances will find their way onto this new car seat. Buy one that has removable and washable pad covers.

- **Comfort.** Babies spend a lot of time in these seats. Find one that looks comfortable to sit in. Look for cloth padding (vinyl seats get very hot and can burn a baby's skin), along with head and back support. Also look for one that is high enough to let your baby see out the window.

■ **Safety.** Look for a label attached to the car seat saying that it meets or exceeds motor vehicle safety standards (sometimes abbreviated as FMVSS 213). Any other kind of seat should never be used in a car.

CARRIER SEAT

This little reclining chair can come in very handy. It lets your son sit up and watch you while you work around the house, and it holds him in a good position for feeding. Unfortunately, this kind of seat can cause severe injury to an infant if it should fall, especially off a high table. Your little bronco rider will soon be kicking and throwing his weight around, so look for an infant seat with a nonskid, wide bottom that will discourage tipping. And never leave your baby alone in an infant seat.

To safely use a carrier seat, follow these safety tips:

☐ The carrier should have a wide, sturdy base for stability.

☐ Stay within arm's reach of the baby when the carrier seat is on tables, counters, or other furniture. Never turn your back. Carrier seats slide more easily on slippery surfaces such as glass tabletops.

☐ If the carrier seat does not already have nonskid feet, attach rough-surfaced adhesive strips to the underside.

☐ Always use the safety belts and keep them snug.

☐ If the carrier seat contains wire supporting devices, which snap on the back, check for security. These can pop out, causing the carrier seat to collapse.

☐ Never place a carrier seat on a soft surface such as a bed or sofa. The carrier seat may tip over and the baby may strangle or suffocate.

☐ Remember that a carrier seat is not always an infant car seat, and should never be used in an automobile unless it is labeled for that purpose.

STROLLERS

Strollers these days are very portable and lightweight, but some don't hold up well when little boys begin to wiggle and turn. When shopping, seek out a sturdy stroller that can hold its ground and won't tip over. Also look for a sunshade and front wheels that pivot. It's also nice to have a model that reclines for comfortable napping.

Here are some tips for choosing a stroller:

■ If you plan to use a stroller before your son can sit up, make sure the stroller fully reclines. With adult supervision, it can double as a portable bed for use indoors or in the park. Just make sure your baby lies on his back and is belted in. The safest belt design is a T-buckle, with a crotch strap and waist belts that connect together.

- Umbrella strollers—lightweight cloth slings with thin metal frames that fold like an accordion—do not provide enough support for newborns and usually don't recline. But they can be fine for short jaunts with a toddler.

- Make sure your stroller has a canopy to block the sun, preferably with a plastic window so you can see the baby. (You won't need the window if your stroller handle reverses so the baby can face you while you push.)

- Check carefully for weight, ease of steering, and ease of folding. Weight it down with twenty or twenty-five pounds and then push it around the store. Try pushing with one hand—you should still be able to steer the stroller in a straight line. Then try folding and unfolding it.

- For stability, the wheelbase should be wide and the seat low in the frame. The stroller should resist tipping backward when you press lightly down on the handles.

- A roomy underseat bin can save your shoulders and back from the strain of carrying heavy bags.

Strolling with Two: Strollers for two come either in tandem style, where one child sits behind the other, or side by side. Not all side-by-sides can fit comfortably through a standard doorway, so check before you buy. Tandems are generally easier to maneuver, especially if you have riders of unequal weight—an infant and a toddler—rather than twins. They're also more compact when folded. But side-by-side transports allow both users to recline more comfortably at the same time. And being side by side may be more fun for them.

> # SCIENCE SAYS
>
> Researchers have found that all healthy newborns act the same. But in the months that follow, boys tend to cry a bit more, sleep less, and are more active than baby girls.

Jogging Strollers: These carriages, also called sport or running strollers, are designed to be pushed as the adult runs or jogs. They are elongated and have three large wheels—one in front and two in back—which make them easier to roll than regular strollers. They're also higher priced—starting at about $150—and too big for indoor use. If you're already a confirmed runner or brisk exercise walker, such a stroller may make sense. If you don't have a good track record on exercise, it may be a waste.

In either case, go slow on getting a jogging stroller: Because of the shaking that comes with higher speed, it's best not to run or jog while pushing your son until he is about one year old. Even then, look for routes that are smooth underfoot.

Baby Boy Toys

A newborn doesn't need many toys, especially the candy-colored stuffed animals they are likely to accumulate as gifts. In fact, it's safer to keep an infant's crib and play area free of toys.

But when you do buy toys for your son, look them over carefully. All toys should have smooth edges and be nontoxic, nonbreakable, and washable. Never give a baby a toy smaller than 1⅝ inches across that can be swallowed (check all parts that may fall off and become a choking hazard). Cut off all ribbons and strings and check all toys occasionally to be sure they are in good repair.

NEWBORN BASICS

Here is a list of toys that are worth considering for your newborn:

- ☐ **Mobile:** A windup or electric mobile visible from the crib can give your son something interesting to look at while lying on his back. Many mobiles also play music. Be sure the mobile is securely fastened, is out of the baby's reach, and not hanging directly over the crib (just in case it falls). Crib mobiles should be removed by the time your child is able to get on hands and knees, usually when he is about five or six months old. A mobile visible from the changing table can also help keep your son amused during diaper changes.

- ☐ **Rattle:** Once your son can grasp something, he'll love rattles, especially if they have parts that spin or otherwise move. But exercise caution when you buy your rattles: Avoid rattles with ball-shaped ends, and check for small ends that could extend into the back of your son's mouth. Take rattles and other small objects out of the crib or playpen when he sleeps. And remember that, like pacifiers, rattles should never be fastened to a cord around a baby's neck.

- ☐ **Padded play mats:** Placed on the floor, often with segments that crinkle or squeak, these are fun for babies who cannot yet crawl.

- ☐ **Floor gyms:** These provide things for babies to grab and bat while they lie on their backs on the floor.

INDOOR SWING

I am convinced that a baby swing saved my sanity. My second son was a cranky baby who calmed only with constant rocking, bouncing, jostling, riding, etc. While visiting a friend who owned a

---

TOYS AND OTHER ITEMS TO AVOID

1. **Pillows, quilts, sheepskins, soft mattresses, or any other kind of soft bedding.** Also, stuffed animals or other soft toys should be kept out of the crib or bassinet. Keeping the baby's sleeping area free of such objects appears to lower the risk of Sudden Infant Death Syndrome (SIDS), which for unknown reasons is higher in baby boys.
2. **Tub seats.** These are intended for use in a bathtub by babies old enough to sit up. But experts advise against using them: They may tempt a parent to leave the baby alone in the tub, which can be extremely dangerous.
3. **Talcum (baby) powder.** If inhaled, it can irritate the lungs.
4. **Latex balloons.** Uninflated or broken, they pose a choking risk.

swing, I found that I could put him in the swing, free up my arms, and get a good twenty minutes of peace. I immediately hurried to the nearest baby supply store, bought him a swing of his own, and brushed my teeth in peace for the first time since his birth! I highly recommend this little lifesaver.

Baby swings are semireclining seats that hang on rigid arms from a four-legged frame. Electric or wind-up versions are available. Babies differ widely in their reaction to swings, so it's best to try them out before buying one, especially because they take up a lot of floor space.

If you do decide to buy a swing, check it carefully for safety. The base should have nonskid, sturdy legs. It must also have a seat belt and crotch restraint to hold his squirmy body in place. I prefer a battery-operated one over the wind-up version because you can reset it without making noise, which could wake your son. An adjustable seat is also a plus so you can recline it for your newborn and raise it as his neck gets stronger.

Ready Or Not

Planning for a little boy is such fun! Tracking his masculine growth through your pregnancy, choosing just the right name, finding a good doctor, and then shopping for the must-have newborn items will fill your B.B. (*before baby*) time with dreams of snakes and snails and puppy dog tails. Then, before you know it, your little boy will be in your arms. That's when the real fun begins!

MY BABY BOY

The best thing about having a son is that it's like watching yourself grow up.

—Dominick Martone
Father of 4-year-old son

Two

Bright Beginnings

Your Boy from Birth Through Three Months

*a*s you welcome your infant boy into your family, this tiny pipsqueak will quickly come to run your life, own your time, and steal your heart. His midnight cries, hungry demands, and endless dirty diapers will certainly tax your patience. But his first smile, adorable coos, and loving stare will take your breath away. You and your son are about to begin a breathtaking roller-coaster ride, so buckle up and hold on. There's nothing in the world like the first three months of parenthood.

The First Moments After Birth

When I first saw my son Joey, I thought he looked like a sailor who'd been in a bar fight. The nurse handed me an eight-pound bruiser with a swollen eye wearing a white skullcap over a large and nearly bald misshapen head. He was not a vision of loveliness—but he was healthy, and he was mine.

Your son may look more appealing than my Joey, but chances are he won't look quite like the baby you've been dreaming of. Instead, he'll look like an infant who has left a watery womb and has been squished through a rather small vaginal opening. Don't be surprised or upset if your baby has any of the following less-than-attractive features, all of which are temporary:

- A cheesy substance (called *vernix caseosa*) that coats the baby's skin to protect it from the amniotic fluid may still be covering parts of his body.

- After a vaginal birth, his head may appear elongated, almost cone-shaped, because it was compressed coming through the birth canal. This will round out within two weeks.

- Fine, downy hair (called *lanugo*) may cover his shoulders, back, forehead, and temples. This will usually be gone by the end of the first week. It will last longer on a premature infant.

- Swollen genitals are common. Due to maternal hormones, your little boy's breasts may also be enlarged. This will disappear in a week to ten days.

- Puffy eyes are usually caused by the eye drops given to infants immediately after birth to prevent infection.

Despite all these less-than-lovely features, there's no doubt your baby will look absolutely beautiful to you and your partner. After all the time and work you've put into bringing this new baby into the world, you can see how truly miraculous this tiny human being really is.

Baby's First Exam

If your son is born in a hospital, there are certain routine procedures that will be performed to assure health and safety. The details vary from hospital to hospital, but the basics remain the same.

THE APGAR EVALUATION

One minute after birth, your son will take his first test called an Apgar evaluation. This rating system is named after its originator, Dr. Virginia Apgar, and is used to evaluate how well a baby adapts to the outside world. Dr. Apgar's name is now used as an acronym for five areas of evaluation:

A: appearance (especially skin color)

P: pulse rate (number of heartbeats per minute)

G: grimace (a baby's response to annoying stimulation, such as a tap or a finger flick to the body)

A: activity (muscle tone is tested through observation and by flexing and feeling the tension in the baby's arms and legs)

R: respiration (how well the baby can breathe and cry on his own)

Each of these factors is rated on a scale of 0 to 2, with 2 being the most desirable score, making for a perfect score of 10. A score of 7 or more indicates the baby is in good condition. A score under 7 indicates the baby is in some kind of distress and needs careful observation or medical attention. This test is repeated five minutes later. A low score is not cause for panic—most babies with low scores turn out to be normal and healthy.

ROUTINE NEWBORN CARE

In between Apgar evaluations, your baby will receive routine newborn care. The doctor or nurse draws a tube of blood from the placental umbilical cord, which is used to identify the baby's blood type and Rh group and may be used for umbilical cord blood banking. At this point, the medical staff or midwife generally will:

- Clear the newborn's nasal passages with a bulb syringe so he can breathe easily.

- Weigh him, measure his length and head circumference, take his temperature, and estimate his gestational age.

- Put antibiotic ointment or drops in his eyes to prevent infection.

- Take his footprints or palm prints for identification, and give both him and his parents ID bracelets or anklets. The nurse will check these IDs each time the baby is brought to you after being out of your sight. (Although some hospitals are now using new blood-typing techniques for this identification, the foot- and fingerprinting routine is still common.)

- Dry him, wrap him in a blanket, put a tiny knitted cap on his head, and perhaps place him in a warmed bassinet (or on the mother's chest), to prevent heat loss. (Newborns cannot regulate their temperatures as well as adults.)

The order in which these things are done vary. If your baby is born in a hospital, these tasks may be done right in the delivery room or in the nursery. Either way, you will probably be given one more chance to hold your baby before you are moved to the recovery room and your son heads to the nursery. Savor and enjoy this moment. It is one you will want to remember forever.

NEWBORN SCREENING TEST (NBU)

Within the first twenty-four to forty-eight hours of your baby's life, he will be given the newborn screening test (NBU), also called the heel-stick test, to screen for various diseases or conditions, such as phenylketonuria (PKU) and congenital hypothyroidism, for which early treatment can prevent death, mental retardation, or physical disability. The test is performed by pricking your baby's heel and putting a few drops of blood on a special filter paper. The paper is allowed to dry and then sent to the newborn screening laboratory where several different tests will be performed.

All states require a newborn screening test, but each state screens for different disorders. Although the NBU is capable of screening for more than fifty disorders, most states screen for less than eight.

You can find out which tests your states screens for through the Save Babies Through Screening Foundation at www.savebabies.org. This site also tells you how you can send a blood sample to a private lab for a complete screening, if you choose.

First Feedings: Breast or Bottle?

One of your first major parenting decisions will be whether to breast- or bottle-feed your son. The choice is not an easy one, but it's yours alone to make. Breast-feeding has gained in popularity mostly because of the medical benefits it offers to the baby. It is known to strengthen the baby's immune system and help prevent allergies, asthma, and SIDS. It also contains substances that help protect a baby from infections until his own immune system matures. It's also true that babies are less likely to have an allergic reaction to breast milk than to cow's milk. And, of course, it is more readily available and cost-efficient than formula.

But many new moms choose to bottle-feed for reasons that are equally important. They may be on medications that could pass through the breast milk and have negative effects on the baby. Working moms might need the convenience of bottle-feeding for the baby's caregivers. They may have a chronic infection such as HIV that may pass to the baby through breast milk. Perhaps they've had breast surgery, thus making breast-feeding difficult. Or they may have the best reason of all: They simply don't want to.

Both breast- and bottle-fed babies grow to be healthy, well-adjusted human beings. Don't feel righteous or guilty about whichever method you use. Just do it because it's best for you, and enjoy every moment you hold your baby in your arms and provide him with both physical and emotional nourishment.

BREAST-FEEDING

Breast-feeding is the most natural thing in the world, but that doesn't mean it comes naturally. Many new mothers have a bit of trouble at first getting their babies to successfully nurse at the breast. So, if this is what you want to do, don't get frustrated and give up too quickly. You and your baby need time and patience to get to know each other and find a system that works best for both of you. The following tips will help get you going in the right direction.

Getting Started: When you lay your son in your arms and offer your breast, your baby may or may not know what to do. Some babies latch on like old pros, while others root around looking for food. If your son is having trouble, give him some help. You can activate the rooting reflex by gently stroking his cheek with your finger or your nipple. This will cause your son to turn toward your breast.

Make sure your baby's mouth encircles the entire nipple area, called the areola, not just the nipple itself. If his mouth encircles the nipple only, you both will be uncomfortable. This can cause your nipples to become sore or even crack, and your son may not get all the milk he needs. Place your nipple in the center of his mouth, with the areola entirely within his lips. Make sure that your breast does not cover his nose and interfere with breathing.

When you begin nursing, it's best to start slowly. Many newborns have very little appetite for the first few days of life, and your breasts need to ease into the process gradually. At first, allow your baby about five minutes on each breast. Over the course of a few days, and depending on the baby's appetite, you can build up to ten minutes per breast and then to fifteen. You should also start nursing on the opposite breast at each feeding. This will keep both breasts evenly producing milk. To break the baby's suction when you're ready to switch breasts, simply place your finger into his mouth, between the nipple and his mouth. And be sure to burp your baby before switching to the other breast and after the feeding is over. (See information later in this chapter for a few tips on burping.)

For the first few days, your breasts will produce a yellowish liquid called colostrum. This doesn't contain much milk, but it is rich in antibodies and protective cells from your bloodstream. These substances help your newborn fight off infections until his own immune system matures. After about five days, the colostrum will diminish and milk will take over.

How Often to Breast-feed: Your baby knows how often he should be fed. He will let you know—loud and clear. Some boys are voracious eaters, and others are quite finicky. In general, breast-fed babies eat more than formula-fed babies because breast milk is less filling than formula. But your baby will determine his own schedule and let you know when he's hungry by fussing, making sucking noises, and by crying.

For the first week or so, your baby will probably need to nurse quite often because his stomach can't hold enough to keep him satisfied for long periods. Every hour is not uncommon. Because nursing can take anywhere from ten to thirty minutes, a hungry infant can take up most of your day.

After a few days, your baby will get the hang of how to suckle just as his appetite kicks in. The regular sucking motions in his face and the gulping sounds will tell you that he is feeding well. You can't measure precisely how much your baby is drinking, but it's comforting to know that your milk supply is determined by how much the baby sucks. If he needs more milk, his increased sucking will prompt your body to produce more milk. This keeps the amount of milk you have and your baby's needs in sync.

Keep your eyes open for signs that your baby is getting enough nutrition. He should be wetting his diaper from five to eight times a day during the first few days and from six to eight times a day afterward. And he should be gaining weight at a rate that satisfies his doctor. When this is the case, you can feel satisfied that he is getting all the nourishment he needs.

Hand-Expressing Breast Milk: Most nursing mothers find that at some point they need to hand-express their milk. I found that when my breasts were overloaded with milk, expressing eased the pain. I also expressed milk into baby bottles to store for later use when a baby-sitter or my husband would be feeding the baby. In any case, expressing milk is an easy process.

Always wash your hands before you begin to express milk. To express by hand, hold a clean container under your breast and place one hand around your breast with the thumb on top. Gently squeeze in a rhythmic fashion, pulling the thumb toward the areola. It's easiest to master this technique when your breasts are full.

You can also express your milk with a manual or electric breast pump. A pump is more efficient if you need to express bottles of milk on a regular basis. Carefully follow the manufacturer's instructions and ask for help from a more experienced friend. Then wash and sterilize the pump immediately after each use or as soon as possible.

Storing Breast Milk: Be very careful about how you store your breast milk. It must always be placed immediately in the refrigerator or freezer. (If you're away from home, store it in an insulated cooler.) It should be used within twenty-four hours if refrigerated, or three months if frozen. If the milk will be stored for a while, put a label on the bottle and date it. If it's to be frozen, don't use a glass bottle or fill it completely because milk expands as it freezes. Refrigerated or frozen breast milk may look different in the bottle because the fat separates from the liquid. It's still good. Just warm the bottle under hot running water or place it in a bowl of hot water. Do not leave it out at room temperature. Also, don't heat the milk in a microwave or on the stovetop. The immune properties of breast milk are heat sensitive, and the uneven heating of a microwave risks scalding the baby. Never refreeze partially used or thawed milk.

Using Breast and Bottle Milk: There may be occasions when you don't have the time or interest in expressing milk, and choose instead to use formula bottle-feeding. Many new moms alternate between the two, but if you decide to do this, you'll need to be careful not to bottle-feed more often than you breast-feed. The bottle's nipple is easier for your baby to suck than your breast, so sucking from a bottle can make your son lazy about sucking from the breast. Also if you offer formula in a bottle too often, the amount of milk your breasts produce will be reduced.

Easing Discomfort: Even with the best intentions and care, sometimes breast-feeding causes breast discomfort and even pain. A common problem is called engorgement. This happens if your breasts are not emptied during each feeding, and it can be very painful. While nursing my first son, I suffered through this without help or guidance. With my second son, a kind and understanding nurse taught me two very helpful methods of reducing the pain of engorgement: 1) expressing milk between feedings to reduce the pressure, and 2) applying warm compresses immediately before feedings to encourage the milk to flow freely. What a relief!

Nursing may make your nipples sore or even cracked until they toughen up. To relieve this discomfort, expose your nipples to the air as much as possible. Pamper them with ultrapurified, medical-grade lanolin, A&D ointment, or vitamin E (squeezed from cap-

BREAST-FEEDING HELP

If you have any trouble, questions, or concerns about breast-feeding, be sure to ask for help. Your doctor may assist you, or you might call in a breast-feeding professional. A lactation consultant at your local hospital, at a woman's health center, or at the La Leche League can help you and your baby adjust to each other. You can contact the La Leche League at 1-800-LALECHE, or *www.lalecheleague.org*.

sules). Wash your nipples with water only. Do not use soaps or re-moistened towelettes. After each feeding, express some milk and massage it onto the nipples. Vary your nursing position so that a different part of the nipple is compressed at each feeding. Hand-express some milk before feeding so that the nipple is easier for the baby to grasp. This pain should last only for about one week. If it continues, talk to your doctor.

BOTTLE-FEEDING

The joy of bottle-feeding is that it allows everyone to have a turn at feeding the new baby—your partner, your son's older siblings, your parents, and your in-laws can all chip in and discover the wonderful feeling of closeness that comes from holding and nour-ishing a newborn. Your baby will probably take to the bottle easily: Bottle nipples are easier for a newborn to grasp onto than the breast. But if your baby doesn't seem interested in eating right away, don't push him. For the first few days, he probably won't be very hungry as he recovers from delivery and adjusts to his new surroundings. Soon, however, his appetite will pick up.

Once you make the choice to bottle-feed, you'll have to decide which kind of formula to use. (Cow's milk straight from the dairy case in your store does not have the nutrients a baby needs in his first year.) Pediatricians recommend a cows' milk–based formula for most babies, and then switching to a soy-based formula if any problems occur. Soy formulas are recommended for infants with a family history of milk allergies.

After deciding on cow's milk or soy-based formula, you have more decisions to make. You can purchase formula in three different forms: ready-to-use, liquid concentrate, and powder. Obviously, the ready-to-use is the easiest form, but it also the most expensive. If you choose concentrate or powder, be sure to follow the mixing and storage instructions to the letter. Diluting formula with the wrong concentration may cause an imbalance in the electrolytes, particularly sodium. Also, the infant can receive too few calories if the formula is too diluted. Make sure the filled bottles are refrigerated until it is time to use them. When traveling, put them in thermal bags to keep them cold. Once you have opened a can of prepared formula or put formula into bottles, use it within forty-eight hours.

Formula should be "served" at room temperature—not warm and certainly not hot. Getting the formula to room temperature is quite an art and very different from the way your mother warmed your bottles. Do not put a bottle in boiling water on the stovetop and do not heat it in the microwave. These methods overheat the food and destroy nutrients. Microwaving is especially dangerous. Because it heats from the inner core out, it is possible for some of the liquid to be scalding hot and you won't know it until the baby drinks it. Shaking the bottle does not reduce the danger from one of these hot spots. Instead, cold or even frozen formula (and stored breast milk, too) should be held under warm running water until it becomes room temperature. Or, you can use a commercial bottle warmer.

Most pediatricians recommend that all baby bottles be sterilized before use until the baby is three months old. You can do this by using a bottle sterilizer found at any baby supply store. Or you can simply use the dishwasher. But be sure to place plastic items on the top shelf and use a dishwasher-safe container to hold small items such as nipples and rings to keep them from getting caught up in the motor. You can also sterilize the bottles by boiling them in a large pot on top of the stove for five minutes. After sterilizing, store the bottles in the refrigerator to keep them bacteria-free.

Once you have all your equipment in hand, it's time to feed your baby. No matter what your well-meaning relatives tell you, feed your newborn on demand. Although he probably won't need to be fed as often as breast-fed babies since formula is more filling, he will still let you know when he is hungry, and you should answer the call. Start with a four-ounce bottle and let your baby decide when he's had enough. Don't try to cajole him into finishing it all if he is clearly full. If you have formula left over, throw it away. Once your baby has sucked from the bottle, it is a breeding ground for bacteria.

FEEDING AND BURPING TIPS

Here are some tips that will help you develop the art of burping and nighttime feedings.

Burping: For you and me, burping comes naturally, but not so for your baby. His gastrointestinal system isn't yet ready to do this work by itself and needs a little help from you. So allow time at every feeding to gently tap him on the back to nudge out a burp or two.

There are several positions you can choose for the burping routine. Try them all and pick the ones that feel most comfortable (but always remember to hold a cloth diaper or towel under the baby's mouth to catch the milk that often comes up with the burp):

- While your son's head is still wobbly, it's easiest to burp him on your shoulder. Rest his head on your shoulder. Use one arm to support his weight under the buttocks, and use the other hand to pat him on the back.

- Sit your son on your lap, supporting his chest and head with one hand. Keeping him tilted slightly forward, pat his back with your other hand.

- Place your son, tummy down, across your thighs. Lower his legs just slightly, supporting his lower half so that his head is higher than his chest. Gently pat his back or rub it in a circular motion.

Breast-fed babies generally burp less than bottle-fed babies because they take in less air, but you'll have to experiment with your child to determine his "burping personality." Some babies are gassier than others and burp often and with vigor. Others give just a few soft burps. Either way, you should routinely burp your baby, between breasts if nursing, or after every two or three ounces of formula if bottle-feeding. Then, even if he has drifted off to sleep, be sure to burp him at the end of a feeding before putting him down to rest.

Nighttime Feedings: Unlike the rest of your household, your newborn does not know the difference between night and day. It's all the same to him and when he's hungry, he's hungry. So until your baby's stomach is large enough to hold more milk—usually when he is about twelve pounds—he will not be able to sleep through the night without waking and crying for food. To establish a nighttime routine that encourages nighttime sleeping, make the night feedings a quiet, quick affair. Change his diaper in a dimly lit room. Then feed, burp, and return him to his bed. No playing, bright lights, or loud talking. The time between feedings should gradually get longer and longer until finally your baby is sleeping through the night.

Comforting Your Crying Baby

All infants cry, especially boys. The first cry after birth fills your newborn's lungs with air and expels any fluid. By two to three weeks of age, infants typically start to develop a type of fussy crying. Most babies have a fussy spell between 6 and 10 P.M. (just when you are apt to feel most frazzled) and sometimes it worsens as the evening goes on. After that, babies cry for innumerous reasons. They cry because they are tired, hungry, bored, wet, uncomfortable, or for no apparent reason at all. Your instinct to go to your baby when he cries is nature's way of making sure your baby learns that he is loved and cared for. So don't let well-meaning family and friends tell you that you'll spoil your infant by picking him up when he cries.

Charles Schaefer, Ph.D., a child psychologist and author of dozens of child-rearing books, assures us when a parent responds quickly to a baby's cry in the first few weeks of life, the newborn feels nurtured. He adds, "For the first six months, it is unlikely you will spoil your baby by swiftly responding to each cry or by surrendering to your impulse to cuddle and comfort. During this time many babies need a great deal of comforting to help ease the transition between intrauterine and independent life. Also, these babies do not have the ability to make the mental connection that enables older children to reason, 'If I cry, I'll get my own way.' Infant cries can, and should, be answered."

TECHNIQUES TO SOOTHE YOUR CRYING SON

Here are a few soothing techniques that Dr. Schaefer recommends for calming a crying baby:

Physical contact: Pick up and cuddle your baby as often as you like. Remember, for the first six months, you will not spoil your baby by giving him too much attention. In fact, babies whose cries are answered promptly in the first three months tend to cry less later on than those whose cries were often ignored. If your baby calms when you carry him, but you can't carry him all day long and get anything else done, use an infant sling to keep him close to your body while you move around.

Rhythmic motion: Many babies stop crying when in motion. Rocking chairs, baby swings, carriage rides, and trips in the car are all modes of movement that calm many wailing babies.

Swaddling: Swaddling in a lightweight receiving blanket often restores a newborn's sense of comfort and closeness. That's why babies are routinely swaddled in hospital nurseries to reduce fearful crying. To swaddle at home, take one corner of a receiving blanket and fold it down six inches. Place the baby on the blanket with his head above the fold. Next, take one side of the blanket and draw it across his body. Fold the bottom section up over his feet, then fold the last section across his body. Finally, turn the swaddled baby onto his stomach. If your son cries harder after swaddling, don't persist. Some babies find it too confining.

Noise: Run the vacuum cleaner near your baby boy to provide a constant humming sound (don't feel you have to actually vacuum!). The static of the radio off channel, the hum of a laundry washer or dryer, or a tape recording of a waterfall, running shower, or heartbeat are all sounds that parents have found will calm a fussy baby.

Comfort sucking: Some babies have strong sucking needs unrelated to their desire for food. Their crying is often controlled by sucking on their fingers, a fist, or a pacifier. (Most babies discontinue this extra sucking around age one.) If you choose to use a pacifier, it should be introduced in the first six to eight weeks, (but wait until breast milk is well established after four to eight weeks if you're breast-feeding to avoid "nipple confusion"). Use pacifiers made from only one piece of rubber, and avoid those that can come apart. Once your son decides on a certain type, it's smart to buy a few extra you can use when one ends up on the floor or is chewed by the dog. Don't coat the pacifier with sugary sweeteners. This habit can cause cavities later on. Never tie the pacifier to a string that is then tied around the child's neck. This could cause strangulation. Take the pacifier away from your son before bed or naps so he doesn't become dependent on it for going to sleep. Pacifiers can gradually be taken away between six to twelve months before your son grows dependent on it.

Singing: Even if you can't carry a tune, singing in a melodic and calm refrain may have magical soothing powers. Some researchers say that certain sounds and melodies, such as lullabies, can provide reassurance for babies by creating a sense of emotional security. So sing to your son often to help him build this association that will provide you with an always-available source of comfort.

Dealing with a fussy baby can be the most exhausting part of early parenting. It can leave you feeling helpless and like a failure, or frustrated and enraged, possibly even setting the stage for child

SCIENCE SAYS

A classic study of sex differences conducted by Howard Moss at the National Institute of Mental Health found some interesting differences in male and female infants and the way their mothers reacted to them. This study of thirty first-time moms found that at age three weeks, baby boys fussed more, cried more, and were more difficult to calm, while baby girls were often more alert, more responsive to efforts to calm them, and slept an average of one hour longer every twenty-four hours. This extra fussing by the boys caused their moms to hold them more, to move and stimulate them more, and in general to give them more of their attention. The baby girls, who seemed more mature and less in need of help to become calm or to remain alert, received less holding, moving, and stimulation.

abuse. If there's no help at hand and you feel at the end of your rope, it's better to put your crying baby in a safe place and leave the room, rather than risk shaking or otherwise hurting him.

Far better to get some relief before the crying pushes you to the edge. If a partner can't help, ask a relative to pitch in or hire someone for a few hours a day and get out of the house. Join a mothering center or parenting group; oftentimes the support of other parents—or honest discussion and sympathy between you and your partner—is all you need to get through these tough weeks. Try to take advantage of those times when the baby is asleep and at rest. Remember, as my mother told me time and time again, this too shall pass. (And she was right!)

Getting Your Son to Sleep

You may be baffled by how your infant son seems to have no concept of night or day. Darkness and daylight will likely mean nothing to him. While you probably like to sleep through the night, you'll soon discover that babies have other plans for the nighttime hours.

INFANT SLEEP SCHEDULE

Your newborn's sleep and wake schedule will likely vary and change over time. At first, he will sleep most of the day (about sixteen out of twenty-four hours) and wake about every three or four hours for a feeding. Then after about a week, he'll begin to spend more time awake and feeding. But it's still too early to set up any kind of sleep or feeding schedule. An infant's stomach is too small to hold enough food to last for long stretches between feedings.

From one to two months of age, infants spend more daytime hours awake, taking in the world around them. Still, most babies this age need at least two one- to three-hour naps every day—one in the morning and one after lunch. If your baby sleeps longer than three or four hours during daytime naps, wake him up so he will be sleepy at bedtime. At this age, many infants begin to skip at least one nighttime feeding. You can encourage a longer stretch between nighttime feedings by letting your son cry and fuss a bit before running to the rescue. Very often babies awake at night (as we all do) and just need a few minutes of fussing to settle back down and fall asleep again. Give your baby a chance to learn how to self-soothe. You'll be glad you did when he is able to put himself back to sleep without your help over the next year.

At this time, you can emphasize the differences between night and day by keeping your son's sleeping room dark at night and doing the necessary feeding and changing in a quick, quiet way. Don't talk, play, or turn on the lights. During the day, let the sunshine in, let the noise and bustle level stay higher, and play and talk with your baby whenever he is awake. Unless your newborn is particularly sensitive to noise, it pays to keep daytime noise levels normal even when he is napping. That way, he'll get used to snoozing through ringing phones and normal conversation.

By six weeks, babies tend to be sleeping longest in the evening, usually for three to five hours, and this trend becomes stronger as the months pass. If you feed him at 10 or 11 P.M., you may even be able to sleep until dawn. At about three months, most bottle-fed babies no longer need feedings at night, even though they may en-

WHEN YOU'RE SERIOUSLY SLEEPY

Despite all the kidding, long-term sleep deprivation for parents or other caretakers can be very unpleasant. It can also be dangerous, leading to accidents at home and in the car, marital tension, and even child abuse when overtired parents lash out at a crying child. The effects of going without sleep tend to be cumulative, building up over months. Take them seriously. Especially in those first few weeks, remember the number-one rule of parent preservation: Sleep when your baby sleeps. Or, if you can't sleep, at least lie down and rest.

joy them. Breast-fed babies usually reach that point a little later, perhaps five or six months.

By three months, your son will be ready to have a more formal sleep schedule. You can begin to put him down at the same time every day for naps and bedtime. Remember to put him to sleep while he's still awake and not feeding. If you feed your baby to sleep, he will need you to do it again and again every time he wakes in the middle of the night. Once he learns to associate feeding with sleeping, it will be hard to break the habit and he will want to suck in order to fall asleep every time. Eventually he'll find he can't put himself back to sleep without a feeding (or the pacifier!). This is also bad for his developing teeth. When the teeth begin to break through at about four months, bedtime feedings make cavities far more likely because the liquid pools around the teeth as a baby sleeps. So after feeding, wake your son, burp him, then put him down so he learns how to put himself to sleep without a feeding. If you do this, most likely your baby will sleep through the night by twelve to sixteen weeks.

SHARING THE FAMILY BED

It's the middle of the night and your baby is crying for a feeding. "Why not," you wonder, "let him sleep in my bed so I don't have to keep getting up?" There are many parents who strongly support the idea of having a family bed and the emotional advantages they feel it engenders. On the other hand, there are many who see this arrangement as both an intrusion of privacy and a dangerous situation for the baby.

In my case, I begrudgingly shared our bed with my middle son because he was a nighttime screamer who would quiet down for longer periods when nestled between me and my husband. It was to be a temporary solution to my own need for more sleep. Three years later, when my baby daughter arrived, I was still waiting for my son to be ready to move back into his own bed—he had no intention of moving over for his little sister. Needless to say, the family bed did not work well for me!

The final decision on whether or not to bring your baby into your bed is entirely up to you. But if you decide to make room for your squiggly infant (even if it's just for the feeding) keep these safety tips in mind:

☐ Remove all pillows and comforters. Your son can't push them out of the way if they get pulled over his face while you sleep. Also, don't bring a baby into your bed if you sleep on

> ## WHEN TO CALL THE DOCTOR
>
> If your baby seems overly irritable and cannot be soothed, or is diffi-
> cult to rouse from sleep and seems uninterested in feeding, speak to
> your doctor. Chances are everything is fine, but it's worth getting
> medical guidance.

a waterbed, feather bed, or sheepskin. They, too, can cause suffocation.

☐ Don't bring your son into your bed if you are under the in-fluence of alcohol, medications, or other drugs. You will not hear his cry if you roll over on him and suffocate him. (Sadly, it has happened.)

☐ Be sure your son can easily sleep on his back to avoid SIDS.

☐ Don't overbundle your son. He will have your body heat as well as his own. Overheating is one suspected cause of SIDS.

☐ Put your son in the middle of the bed so he can't roll off. (Even newborns work their way across a bed as your own body shifts positions during the night.)

Postpartum Disorders

In recent years, the often-ignored and misunderstood mood imbal-ance postpartum depression (PPD) has become a household phrase. As you recover from the birth of your baby, you should be aware of the symptoms of postpartum depression. But also understand that there are varying degrees of this mood disorder.

POSTPARTUM BABY BLUES

What some call "postpartum blues" or "baby blues" is a mild form that the American College of Obstetricians and Gynecologists says affects about 70 to 85 percent of new moms. Within the first three days after giving birth, feelings of fatigue, nervousness, confusion, detachment from the baby, and anxiety accompanied by frequent bouts of crying set in. Most medical experts agree that these blues are caused by dramatic physiological changes that occur in hormonal levels after birth. (Levels of estrogen and progesterone drop as much as tenfold!) Social factors such as lack of family support and psychological factors like marital tension can also play a role in causing and/or aggravating this mild form of PPD. Baby blues generally go away without any form of treatment within a week or two.

POSTPARTUM DEPRESSION

Postpartum depression (which affects about 10 percent of new mothers) is more intense and lasts longer than the blues. It can develop at almost any time up to one year after childbirth, but most often appears sometime between the second week and third month after birth. Typically, it can last anywhere from several weeks to several months.

Moderate PPD is apparently rooted in negative social and psychological factors, including the daily stresses of parenting, feelings of isolation, a colicky infant, chronic lack of sleep, and marital tensions. It is best treated with professional help because it often responds well to a combination of antidepressant medication and cognitive therapy that teaches you to better cope with the stress of parenthood.

If you have feelings of moderate PPD, you shouldn't ignore them or let them go untreated. Dr. Schaefer says that if a month or two go by and you are not yet feeling any enthusiasm about motherhood, or if you still aren't experiencing normal eating and sleeping patterns, you should call your doctor or the support group (see "Warning Signs of Postpartum Depression," page 66). In rare cases, the symptoms persist and greatly increase in severity. This may indicate the onset of the most serious form of PPD called postpartum psychosis.

POSTPARTUM PSYCHOSIS

Postpartum psychosis (PPP) affects only about one in one thousand women and most often occurs during the first four weeks after delivery. Women with PPP are severely impaired and may have paranoia, mood shifts, or hallucinations and delusions that frequently focus on the infant's dying or being demonic. These hallucinations often command the woman to hurt herself or others. This condition requires immediate medical attention and, usually, hospitalization.

> ## CARING FOR SYMPTOMS OF
> ## POSTPARTUM MOOD DISORDER

In the book *Raising Baby Right*, which I co-wrote with Dr. Schaefer, he suggests that if you are feeling the symptoms listed in the box "Warning Signs of Postpartum Depression," you should follow these two steps:

1. **Take care of yourself.** Learn to recognize your overload factors and avoid them. If you feel you can't keep the house clean *and* take care of the baby, let the house go. If the visits of family and friends send you into a tizzy as you try to be a good host and cater to the needs of your newborn, take the phone off the hook and disconnect the doorbell. Get a sitter and make time to go for a walk, take a warm bath, or nap. Stay alert to the signs of depression and talk to your doctor if you start to feel them. Take care of yourself first and foremost. If you do this, you'll have the emotional and physical strength you need to take care of all your other responsibilities.

2. **Seek support.** Don't try to handle your negative feelings alone. These feelings do not mean you are a bad mother, nor do they in any way indicate that you can't handle motherhood. They are very common feelings shared, to some degree, by approximately eight out of ten new mothers—the majority of whom turn out to be wonderful parents.

   Talk to your partner. He can't understand your feelings and actions unless you explain what's going on. His emotional support is very important to your ability to overcome your problem. Ask him or her for that help.

Talk to other mothers. Sharing your frustrations lessens their load, and hearing about similar experiences will take away some of the horror and mystery of this trying period.

Talk to your doctor. He or she can help you determine the level of your depression and decide on a treatment plan that will give you back your enthusiasm for parenthood.

Postpartum depression is very treatable, so you should get medical help promptly if you are depressed most of the time for two weeks or more.

WARNING SIGNS OF POSTPARTUM DEPRESSION

The American College of Obstetricians and Gynecologists warns that women with postpartum depression have feelings of being overwhelmed, are unable to cope with daily tasks, and feel guilty about not being a good enough mother. Other symptoms include:

deep sadness	crying spells
apathy	irritability
lack of appetite	intense anxiety
highly impaired concentration and decision-making	inability to sleep
	irrational behavior

Health and Hygiene in the Early Weeks

In the first three months, there's so much to think—and worry—about. Right from the start, you'll need to care for the health and hygiene of your son. Top on the list of things to do will be caring for his penis (especially if he's been circumcised) and umbilical cord stub, tending to the endless task of diapering, and, of course, bathing.

CIRCUMCISION DECISIONS

About 1.2 million newborns are circumcised each year. Lately the practice has come under scrutiny by parents who question the necessity for this procedure. Circumcision for other than religious reasons is a relatively recent phenomenon in the United States. It began in the late nineteenth century and peaked in the 1960s when 90 percent of newborn males were circumcised. Interestingly, the procedure is not common elsewhere. In Canada, the rate is 17 percent and in Britain, 5 percent. Elsewhere in Europe, South America, and in non-Muslim Asia, the procedure is quite rare. So why are so many American males being circumcised?

There are many doctors who believe that circumcision helps prevent urinary tract infections, penile cancer, and sexually transmitted diseases, including HIV. But there are others in the medical community who believe that the risks of infection and cancer are low even without the procedure, and its effects on the transmission of sexually transmitted diseases are unclear. But they worry about complications that can occur with any surgery and feel that there is not enough sound reason to recommend routine circumcision.

That leaves the final decision regarding circumcision up to you.

CARE OF THE PENIS

In a newborn, the uncircumcised penis is usually completely covered by the foreskin. The foreskin remains attached to the tip of the penis in infancy so you shouldn't attempt to pull it back to clean underneath. (By about the age of five years, the foreskin almost always has become retractable. At this point the boy can be taught to slide the foreskin back and clean the tip of the penis.) The opening in the foreskin should be large enough to allow the infant to urinate with a forceful stream. Consult the doctor if your son's urine only dribbles out.

If you decide to have your son circumcised, immediately after the circumcision, the tip of the penis is usually covered with gauze coated with petroleum jelly. This dressing will come off when the baby urinates. It is probably not necessary to apply a new dressing as long as the area is gently wiped clean with soap and water when the diaper is changed. Healing is rapid and any redness or irritation of the penis should subside within a few days. Complications are quite rare, but if the redness or swelling increases or if pus-filled blisters form, infection may be present and you should call the doctor immediately.

CARE OF THE UMBILICAL CORD

When the baby's umbilical cord is cut at the time of delivery, a small stump attached to the navel area remains. This umbilical cord stump

WHEN TO CALL THE DOCTOR

You should consult your son's doctor if the navel area becomes reddened, is oozing puss, or if a foul odor or discharge develops.

does not need exceptional care. Just keep it clean and dry. To keep the stump clean, dab some rubbing alcohol on a sterile cotton ball and apply to the area periodically to help prevent infection until the cord stump dries up and falls off, usually in ten days to three weeks. Hold off on submerging the navel area during bathing until this occurs. The withering cord stump will change color, from yellow to brown or black. This is normal, so don't worry.

Keep your son's diaper off the stump to avoid chafing. Most newborn disposable diapers now have an area cut out in the umbilical cord area to keep it from rubbing against the cord. But if you do not have this kind of diaper, simply fold the type you have—whether disposable or cloth—below the navel area. If your son's diaper or clothing sticks to the stump, do not pull it off. First wet the area with warm water to loosen the grip, then gently lift apart.

DIAPERING 101

If you've never diapered a baby before, the task can be intimidating. But don't worry. This is one skill that you get to practice over and over again, making you a pro in no time. The people who count this kind of thing say that you're likely to change your son's diaper three thousand times! So don't be afraid; jump right in.

Think safety first. Always have everything you need at hand *before* you begin diapering. You cannot leave your son alone on a changing table for even a second while you turn away to reach for a new diaper. Have at hand warm water and sterile cotton or a clean face cloth, diaper ointment, and a clean diaper. Also, make sure your baby is on a secure surface and keep one hand on him at all times. (Even newborns move in unpredictable ways.)

To begin diapering, lay your son on his back. If you are right-handed, his feet should be to your right side, his head to your left. If you are left-handed, place his feet to your left and his head to your right. This puts your dominant hand near the diaper area and free to do all the work. Unfasten the soiled diaper. Then holding both his ankles securely in one hand (the non-dominant hand that is closest to his head), lift your son's legs and bottom up off the surface. With your other hand remove the soiled diaper and wash his bottom.

You'll be surprised to see that your newborn's bowel movements (BMs) do not look like yours. Watery, greenish, or yellow-colored BMs are perfectly normal in infants for about the first three months. You might see small, hard "rabbit pellets" if your son is constipated; if he has diarrhea, it may look like water. Black, tarlike BMs are not healthy and should be reported to the baby's doctor.

If the diaper is heavily soiled, you can wipe his bottom with the clean part of the diaper to remove some excess. Then wash the bottom and genital area with a sterile cotton ball or washcloth dipped in warm water. Commercial baby wipes are too harsh for a newborn's skin, so stick with water for the first month or two.

At first, your newborn will require very frequent changes. But after a few weeks, he will require fewer changes, and you'll be able to better get organized into a routine. Some babies move their bowels as they are eating, others wait until after, and still others will be soiled before they even begin a feeding. Once you know when your baby is likely to have a BM, you'll know when to be prepared with clean diapers.

Cloth Diapers: If you opt to use cloth diapers rather than disposables, and do not use a diaper cleaning service, you must be very careful to clean them thoroughly. When you remove a soiled diaper from your baby, empty any bowel movement into the toilet immediately. Then put the diapers into a diaper pail partially filled with water. Wash the diapers in a separate wash load with a mild soap or detergent.

Diapering Baby Boys: Having a boy adds a degree of challenge to the diapering process. Keep this information in mind as you begin to diaper your new son:

- If he has been circumcised, his penis will be red and raw for a few days afterward. It's important to keep it clean while diapering. Use warm water applied with a sterile cotton ball (not a cosmetic one, which can irritate the skin). Place a piece of gauze pre-smeared with petroleum jelly over the penis tip to keep away irritating urine. Clean the area and reapply a new gauze pad with each diaper change. It should heal in about a week and no additional care will be required beyond routine bathing. During this time, a yellow secretion is a normal sign of healing, but if yellow-crusted sores develop or redness persists beyond one week, an infection may have developed and you should call his doctor.

DIAPERING TIPS

If you're using cloth diapers these quick tips can make the job easier:

- You can help keep the diapers unstained by adding one-half cup of borax per gallon of water to the diaper pail.

- When washing diapers, don't use too much soap or detergent. Too much is hard to rinse out thoroughly and the leftover can irritate a baby's bottom.

- Do not use fabric softener because this reduces the diaper's absorbency.

- Store the diaper pins by sticking them in a bar of soap. You'll always know where they are, and the soap helps the pin slide more easily into the diaper.

- Diapering an uncircumcised boy requires no special attention. At birth, the foreskin is attached to the head of the penis. It eventually separates and the foreskin must then be pulled back for cleaning, but that won't be for a while. The separation happens in half of all boys by the end of the first year. For some boys, however, it may take up to three years. Ask your son's doctor when you can safely retract the foreskin for cleaning. Until then, simply bathe the penis with soap and water, rinsing thoroughly.

- If you're using cloth diapers, fold the cloth to add extra bulk in the front where the urine needs absorbing.

- You might want to keep a cloth over your son's penis whenever the diaper area is exposed. This will protect you from getting sprayed.

Diaper Rash: Babies wear diapers all day long, and even the most conscientious parent will eventually face diaper rash. But the problem can be prevented somewhat by following these guidelines:

- Change diapers often. Be especially quick to remove a diaper soiled by a bowel movement.

- Wrap diapers loosely. The new form-fitting disposables let very little air on your baby's bottom, so try not to put them on too tightly.

- Ease up on vigorous cleanings. Your baby's bottom is delicate. Too much rubbing and/or too harsh soap can be very irritating.

- Change diapering products. If your son's rash keeps coming back, try different diapers, soaps, ointments, powders, etc. He may be allergic to one of these products.

Even with the best preventative tactics, it's likely that your son will occasionally have diaper rash. When that happens, here are some ways to ease the pain:

- ☐ Air out his bottom. If at all possible, let your baby be totally free of a diaper and any ointment for a few hours each day. If that's not possible, cut away the elasticized legs opening of disposable diapers to allow air to circulate. Air is a great healer.

☐ Soak him in a tub of barely warm water. Do not use soap! This adds to the irritation.

☐ Apply diaper ointment liberally. This will help keep urine off his sore bottom.

☐ Do not use baby wipes to clean after each bowel movement. These can be very irritating to sensitive skin.

Most rashes will go away in a few days. But if your son's rash will not heal or is causing fever or loss of appetite, call his doctor. Sometimes severe rashes require antibiotics and medicated ointments.

BATHING

An infant doesn't need much bathing if you wash the diaper area thoroughly during regular changes. In fact, most pediatricians agree that your newborn should only have sponge baths during his first week or two, until the stump of his umbilical cord falls off and the navel heals over. Then, a bath two or three times a week in the first year is sufficient. More bathing may dry out his delicate skin.

When you do give your baby a sponge bath, get yourself prepared before you bring your baby to the water. In the room where you want to bathe him, gather together a basin of warm water, a clean washcloth, mild baby soap, baby shampoo (if needed), and one or two towels or a blanket. To test the water temperature, stick your elbow in. It should feel warm, not hot or cold.

NO DAILY BATHS

When it comes to skin and hair, babies don't have to contend with some of the hygiene issues that adults do: They don't perspire under their arms, they don't work out, and they don't have hair that gets overly greasy! Instead of bathing your baby every day, which can result in dry skin, limit baths to two or three a week. On off days, just wash your baby's face, hands, and diaper area.

Pick a warm room and any surface that's flat and comfortable for you both, such as a changing table, floor, or counter next to the sink. If the surface is hard, lay down a towel or blanket. If your son is not on the floor, use a safety strap or keep one hand on him at all times to make sure he doesn't fall.

Undress your son and wrap him in a towel, exposing only the part of his body you are washing at the moment. First, wash his face with a dampened washcloth without soap. Then wet the cloth again and wash the rest of his body. Pay special attention to creases under his arms, behind his ears, around his neck, and in the genital area. Once you have washed those areas, make sure they are dry.

Into the tub: Once the umbilical cord stump has fallen off and the navel has healed, you can try placing your son directly in the water. His first baths should be gentle and brief. If he seems miserable, go back to sponge baths for a week or two, then try the regular bath again.

Many parents like bathing their newborn in a special baby tub, the sink, or a plastic tub lined with a clean towel. Whatever type of tub you use, fill the basin (before you place him inside) with two inches of warm water, testing it with your elbow. If you're filling the basin from the tap, turn the cold water on first and off last to avoid scalding your son or yourself. Make sure your hot water heater is set no higher than 120° Fahrenheit.

Once you've undressed your son, place him in the water right away so he doesn't get chilled. Use one of your hands to support his head and the other to guide his body in, feet first. Talk gently to him and slowly lower the rest of his body until he's in the tub. Most of his body and face should be well above the water level for safety, so you'll need to pour warm water over his body frequently to keep him warm.

Use a soft cloth to wash his face and hair, shampooing once or twice a week. Massage his scalp gently, including the area over his fontanels (soft spots). Don't worry. You won't hurt him by doing this. When you rinse the soap or shampoo from his head, cup your hand across his forehead so the suds run toward the sides, not into his eyes. If you get soap in his eyes, take a wet washcloth and wipe his eyes with lots of lukewarm water until the suds are gone and he open his eyes again. When your baby comes out of the bath, wrap him in a towel, making sure his head is covered. Baby towels with hoods are very handy for this move.

The most important rule of baby bathing is this: If you have forgotten something—or need to answer the phone or door during the bath—take your son with you. *Never leave a baby alone in a bath.*

After a while, you and your son may find that bath time is the best time of day. It's a chance for both of you to enjoy the soothing effects of water and to give each other your undivided attention.

Early Medical Care

Your newborn son is far sturdier than he appears, though he does need you to look after his health and give him continued medical care and checkups.

ROUTINE AT-HOME HEALTH CARE

Keeping your newborn healthy is a top priority in the first few months. The best way to do that is to limit his exposure to illness. The immune system of newborns is less mature and developed than that of older children and adults. Because of this, it's a good idea to limit your son's exposure to visitors in the first weeks.

Ask your child's doctor when it is appropriate to take him into crowds, such as a trip to the mall. Stuffy stores and crowded spaces are breeding places for germs, so it's usually best to stay far away for the first few weeks. Also, if friends or relatives have a cold or an infection, ask them to delay visiting until they are better. If you, your partner, or a sibling becomes ill, of course it is harder (if not impossible) to keep your son from being exposed. But, if possible, limit the sick person's contact with him so this person doesn't cough in his face or kiss him until recovered. Everyone in the household should practice good hygiene, by washing his or her hands thoroughly before touching the baby.

SUNBURN ALERT

An infant is extremely sensitive to sun and sunburn during the first six months. Therefore, keep him out of direct and reflected sunlight (such as off concrete, water, or sand), especially during the peak sunlight hours of 10 A.M. to 4 P.M. Dress him in lightweight, light-colored clothing with a bonnet or hat to shade his face. If he's lying or sitting in one place, make sure it is in the shade and adjust his position when the sun moves. If you must take him into sunlight, definitely use sunblock to protect his skin

ROUTINE MEDICAL CHECKUPS

All infants need ongoing professional medical care, and it's your responsibility to make sure your son sees his doctor on a regular basis.

According to Stephen Muething, M.D., section director of clinical services at Cincinnati Children's Hospital Medical Center, babies generally receive routine medical checkups twice in their first three months: often at one week and then again at two months. To get the most out of these visits, Dr. Muething recommends that you prepare in advance. "I'm a big believer in the assertive parent," he says. "Write down your questions and concerns. You're probably going to be feeling tired. The baby may start crying during the exam. The doctor may be rushed, and with all that's going on, it's hard to remember what information you want to take home with you. Don't just go with the doctor's agenda during the visit and remain passive. Families who get more bang for their buck go in saying, 'This is what we need to know at this visit: We have these three questions and we need to talk to you about this.' "

One-week exam: When you take your son for his first medical checkup, use it as an opportunity to learn more about his health and to begin to get to know his doctor.

Either before or during this visit, you'll be asked a long list of questions that will help the doctor better care for your newborn.

The first group of questions will pertain to prenatal history. The doctor may ask questions such as: What was the pregnancy like? Did you have any health problems? Did you get regular prenatal care? Did you take any medications or over-the-counter drugs? Did you drink alcoholic beverages (including beer or wine) and if so, how much? Did you smoke during pregnancy? Did you use any drugs like marijuana or cocaine? (Don't feel insulted by any of these questions. You should doubt the competency of the doctor who *doesn't* ask them.)

You will then be asked about the birth experience. The doctor may ask: Was the baby full-term or premature? If premature, how many weeks early was he born? How much did the baby weigh? Were there any signs of fetal distress during birth? How was the baby delivered (vaginally, by cesarean, with forceps, or with a vacuum extractor)? How long did labor and delivery take? At birth, did the baby need any help breathing? Did he need to spend any time in a special care unit or the neonatal intensive care unit (NICU)? Did he need treatment for jaundice? How long did he stay in the hospital? Did the doctor who examined him in the hospital tell you of any problems? (If you did not give birth to your baby—if he is adopted or in foster care—the doctor will ask you for any information you have about his birth and prenatal history, and about the biological family's medical history.)

The doctor may also want to know about the baby's life at home. He may ask: How is he doing with the main newborn activities—eating, sleeping, pooping, and peeing? When does he sleep and for how long? Where does he sleep? Do you always put him to sleep on his back, the safest position to prevent SIDS? How many wet diapers does he have each day? How often does he have bowel movements? How is the rest of the family doing? Do you feel comfortable taking care of the baby? Are you and your partner having any conflicts over his care? Are you getting any sleep? How is your mood (happy, elated, stressed, depressed, etc.)? Do you get support from family, friends, or hired caregivers? And so on.

With this information in mind, the doctor will turn his attention to your baby and give him a complete going over. He will double-check to make sure that nothing unusual was missed in the hospital such as a cleft lip, ear abnormalities, or heart murmur. He will also check your baby's bilirubin level to see if he has jaundice. (See "Jaundice" on page 85 for more information.)

The doctor will then begin the physical exam. He or the nurse will weigh the baby and measure his length and head circumference. He may also take your son's vital signs (heart rate, breathing rate, and temperature) and record them on his medical chart. Then the doctor will give your son a thorough physical.

☐ He listens to the baby's heart and lungs with a stethoscope.

☐ He examines the baby's abdomen. He checks to see that the umbilical cord is not getting infected and that the navel (belly button) is healing well. A few days after the cord has fallen off, normal skin should have grown over the navel. If not, the doctor may swab on some silver nitrate to help it heal. He then feels the baby's abdomen to be sure that it is soft, not tender, and has no unexpected masses. While feeling your baby's belly, he checks that his liver, kidneys, and spleen are not enlarged.

☐ He makes sure the baby's hip joints are developing properly. He looks to see that the skin creases on both thighs are the same. Then he pushes the baby's hips down into the table and rotates them, moving the knees outward and down toward the table. If he feels the joints slip, the baby may have a condition called developmental dysplasia of the hip.

☐ He checks the baby's femoral pulses (the pulses between the thigh and the abdomen) to make sure there is good blood flow from the heart to the lower half of the body.

☐ He examines the baby's legs, feet, and overall skin color and condition.

☐ He examines the genitals. He checks that both testes have descended and are in the scrotum. (Look for more on undescended testes later in this chapter.) If your baby boy was circumcised, he checks how that is healing.

☐ He examines the head, noting the shape and feel of the fontanels, or the "soft spots" where the bony plates of the skull have not yet joined.

☐ He checks the suck and gag reflexes. (Your baby should suck when something is placed in the front of his mouth and gag when something is placed toward the back of the throat.)

☐ He examines the eyes to see if they are aligned, checks the position of the ears, and looks inside the eardrums.

At this first visit, the doctor will also focus on your son's feeding. He may ask questions such as: How often does he eat? How long does he nurse at the breast, or how much formula does he take? Have you had any nursing problems? Does he seem satisfied after eating? The doctor will also want to make sure that you're comfortable with your chosen method of feeding, be it breast or bottle.

Two-month visit. In addition to a thorough physical, the doctor may also check your son's reflexes at the two-month visit. Some that may be checked include:

☐ The startle (or Moro) reflex. A loud or sudden noise should make your son stretch his arms and legs out, then draw his arms back into his chest.

☐ The step and place reflex: If held as if he's "standing" on a flat surface, your son will lift his legs as if taking steps. If held so the tops of his feet are dragging against a surface (such as the underside of a table), he'll lift his legs as if to step up onto the surface.

☐ The Babinski reflex. If the sole of the foot is stroked from heel to toe, your son stretches his toes up and fans them out (the opposite of what older children and adults do, which is to curl their toes down).

The doctor also checks how your son is developing. He does this by asking you questions, watching the baby, and interacting with him. He may check his development while doing the physical exam or he may do a developmental exam separately. He is checking things such as:

☐ Does he watch people's faces and can he make eye contact?

☐ Does he move both arms and both legs equally?

☐ Does he make any sounds besides crying?

☐ Does he follow an object with his eyes as it moves from the side of his visual field to the midpoint?

☐ If placed on his stomach, can he raise his head? If so, how far?

Again, at the two-month checkup, be sure to come prepared to ask questions and tell the doctor about your concerns. Most doctor visits last less than twelve minutes, so being organized can help you get the most out of that time.

PHONE CALLS TO THE DOCTOR

Many doctors have phone hours when you can call with routine questions. In some practices, a nurse or nurse practitioner may handle most of these calls unless you specifically want or need to talk to the doctor. Don't hesitate to call with your concerns, no matter how small they may seem. Of course, if you suspect your son is ill and may need prompt attention, don't wait for phone hours—call your doctor immediately.

Calls for Illness: Any sign of illness in a baby less than three-months old requires immediate attention because a newborn's condition can quickly deteriorate. The younger and smaller the baby, the more vulnerable he is.

Even a serious illness in a newborn may have seemingly minor symptoms, such as fussiness, drowsiness, or fever over 100.5°. If you are in doubt about a young baby's health, it is better to err on the side of caution even if means taking him to the emergency room. It is far better to ask for advice than to self-diagnose or -medicate.

Calls for Emergencies: If your son has any of the following conditions, call the doctor immediately or, depending on the child's condition, call 911 or go to the emergency room:

- trouble breathing
- head injury with loss of consciousness, vomiting, or blue or pale skin color
- bleeding that won't stop
- poisoning
- seizures
- sudden loss of energy or ability to move

- high fever

- bloody urine

- bloody diarrhea

- any fever or abnormal behavior in a child under 3 months

COMMON INFANT HEALTH CONCERNS

In the first three months of life, your infant son will give you plenty to wonder and worry about. The health concerns that many parents fret over include jaundice, undescended testicle, hernia, colic, and SIDS. Here are the facts.

Jaundice. This condition causes yellowing of the skin and whites of the eyes, and is quite common in newborns. It is caused by a buildup in the blood of bilirubin, a substance produced by the nor-

IMMUNIZATION SCHEDULE

At your son's routine medical checkups, he will receive a series of immunization shots from birth to eighteen months. Be sure to follow your doctor's instructions on when to bring your baby in for his immunizations and check out the current recommended immunization schedule at the website of the American Academy of Pediatrics at www.aap.org, or the Centers For Disease Control at www.cdc.gov/nip/acip.

mal breakdown of red blood cells. Usually bilirubin passes through the liver and is excreted as bile through the intestines, but sometimes it builds up faster than a newborn can pass it from his body.

If bilirubin levels begin to climb too high after birth and if the baby is born in a hospital, treatment with phototherapy begins right away before dangerous levels are reached. The baby is placed unclothed under blue or broad-spectrum white light until bilirubin levels fall. The light alters the bilirubin so that it is more rapidly excreted by the liver. If the baby is already home when jaundice emerges, he may be treated at home with a portable light unit or he may need to return to the hospital.

Undescended Testicle. Shortly before a boy is born, his testicles descend through a tunnel or passageway in the groin (called the inguinal canal) from the abdomen into the scrotum. When a testicle doesn't make the move, the condition is called cryptorchidism. Usually an undescended testicle will come down on its own during the first six months of life. In the remaining cases (less than 1 percent of full-term boys) surgery is sometimes needed to bring the testicle down. The operation, called orchiopexy, is usually done on an outpatient basis when the child is about one year old, and most children feel well enough to be active soon afterward. This prompt treatment is needed because the testicle's ability to produce sperm can be permanently damaged if it remains in the abdomen, which is hotter than the scrotum. An undescended testicle is also more vulnerable to injury.

Hernia. A type of hernia that occurs up to ten times more often in boys is called an *inguinal hernia*. This is a bulge of soft tissue through a weak spot in the abdominal wall in the groin area. Inguinal hernias can occur in one or both sides of the groin at the same time or at different times. They are more common in boys because these abdominal-wall cavities are often created by testicular development.

Surgery is necessary to repair an inguinal hernia, so call a health professional if:

☐ Your son has a definite lump in the groin area.

☐ Your son has a tender bulge in the groin or scrotum, even if the bulge disappears when lying down.

Pyloric stenosis: It is normal for babies to spit up small amounts from their feedings, but repeatedly vomiting large amounts is not normal. It may be a symptom of pyloric stenosis, which affects males four to eight times more often than females. Pyloric stenosis is a condition in which the connection between a baby's stomach and small intestine (pyloric sphincter) gradually swells and blocks food from entering his intestine. This causes him to forcefully vomit most or all of his feedings. Pyloric stenosis can occur anytime between birth and five months of age. However, it most commonly develops about three weeks after birth.

Vomiting caused by pyloric stenosis usually starts gradually and gets worse over time. Once pyloric stenosis begins to develop, there is no way to stop the progression of the condition. As the opening between the stomach and intestine becomes tighter, he will vomit more frequently and more forcefully (also known as projectile vomiting). This condition must be treated with routine surgery to widen the channel between the stomach and the intestine. You should call your son's doctor if he has vomited most or all of his food for two feedings in a row.

COLIC

My middle son was a crier—actually, more of a screamer. From the moment of birth, he made it known that he had arrived, though I was never exactly sure what he needed. There was no stopping the tears, no pleasing him, and no relief for me.

It was of some consolation when the pediatrician gave these crying jags a name: colic. He told me that colic is the extreme end of normal crying behavior in a baby between three weeks and three months of age. I quickly learned that in a baby with colic, the crying lasts longer (more than three hours a day), occurs more often (more than three days a week), and is more intense than expected for the baby's age.

I also learned that it is very difficult to console a baby once an episode of colic has started. Your son may appear to be in pain, flailing and screaming, with tense legs drawn up to his belly. But his crying is not due to hunger, a wet diaper, or other visible causes, and he cannot be calmed down.

So why do colicky babies cry so much? Your parents and grandparents may tell you that colic is caused by gastrointestinal problems such as stomach pain due to gas in the intestine and digestive problems such as milk allergies. But modern medicine now says it is not a disease. Today, evidence suggests that colic is due to the baby's temperament and an inability to regulate crying. A baby's temperament may make him extremely sensitive to the environment, and he reacts to any changes by crying. A baby's nervous system is immature, which results in him being unable to calm down once the crying starts.

Although the parents of every crying baby suspect colic, only about 10 to 30 percent of babies actually cry long and often enough to wear the medical term. Fortunately, babies with colic grow and develop normally, and they are just as likely as other children to be healthy and happy. (It's my own sanity I came to worry about!) In most cases, it goes away on its own in about three months.

Dealing with colic. If your baby's doctor has confirmed that he is perfectly healthy and has no physical reason for his frequent crying, the best you can do is to use a trial-and-error method to find ways to calm his screams.

When he is fed, rested, and diapered, you can try any of the calming strategies mapped out earlier in this chapter. In addition, you might find, as I did, that there is peace in constant motion: walk or rock him; put him in the swing or infant seat; sing songs and dance around the room; place him across your lap on his belly and rub his back while you sway your legs; put him in the car or stroller and give him a ride. Really, anything is worth a try.

Often, despite your best efforts, your colicky baby will continue to cry. When that happens, it's *sooooo* frustrating—enough to make you wonder why you ever thought it would be a good idea to have this baby in the first place. That's when it's time to step back and try to salvage your sanity. Here are a few strategies that worked for me:

Don't blame yourself. There are far too many factors involved to take sole responsibility for colic. Neither you nor your partner should let these periods of crying convince you that you are inadequate parents. While your infant is wailing, remind yourself over and over again that this is not your fault. You have done nothing to cause the crying. You are a good parent.

Expect the crying. If your baby has colic, one thing you can count on is that he won't skip an evening of screaming. Don't plan to have dinner or visitors or quiet conversations during his usual crying time. Plan to spend the colicky period practicing soothing tactics.

Take a break. You can't stand on your eyelashes to calm your son for three hours on end without becoming overwhelmed with anger. You will need time out. Encourage your partner to share the responsibility by taking turns using soothing tactics, and arrange for a sitter on a regular basis so you can get away from your son. As odd as it sounds, the growth of a positive relationship with a colicky baby may depend on how often you can get away from him to calm down by taking a walk, visiting a friend, or sitting in a bath.

Don't forget the colic is temporary. Like pregnancy, colic, too, is a stage of growth and development that will end. Typically the crying periods peak at six weeks of age and then taper off by three months. Eventually, all children grow out of colic.

Remember that the crying will not hurt your son. This is perhaps the hardest lesson of all to learn because it is so difficult for parents to let their babies cry, even when it is apparent that nothing is going to stop the crying.

SUDDEN INFANT DEATH SYNDROME

For all parents, Sudden Infant Death Syndrome (SIDS) is an unspeakable fear. Because SIDS is the leading cause of death in the post-neonatal period (one month to one year) and is more likely to strike boys than girls, it may be an especially nagging worry for you. SIDS is that mysterious syndrome in which seemingly healthy babies go to sleep and are found dead—for no apparent reason. That, of course, is frightening.

By definition, SIDS is the sudden death of an infant under one year that is unexplained even after a thorough investigation. The American Academy of Pediatrics says that the occurrence of SIDS is rare during the first month of life, increases to a peak between two and four months old, and then declines.

The good news is that SIDS is relatively rare, striking fewer than 3,000 babies a year, and getting rarer. Rates have declined by 50 percent since 1992 when the American Academy of Pediatrics began to recommend that healthy babies be put to sleep on their backs.

Why should sleeping position make such a difference? Some speculate that when babies sleep on their stomachs, the air they exhale may get trapped in folds of bedding. The babies then may rebreathe this air, which is low in oxygen and high in carbon dioxide. Rising levels of carbon dioxide should wake a baby, who might cry, cough, or move his head enough to get more fresh air. But some babies fail to wake, perhaps because their brain function is immature or abnormal.

If this theory is correct, it may describe just one of several causes of the mysterious deaths. Researchers have identified other factors, besides stomach sleeping, that seem to increase the risk of

SIDS. These include: sleeping on a soft surface, overheating, smoking during pregnancy by the mother, exposure to smoke after birth, late or no prenatal care, premature birth or low birth weight, and simply being male.

Based on these findings, the American Academy of Pediatrics and other authorities suggest some ways likely to reduce the risk of SIDS:

- Healthy newborns, including most premature newborns, should be put to sleep on their backs.

- Make sure that all caregivers understand that the baby must sleep on his back. Stomach-sleeping used to be standard in the United States, and many grandparents and baby-sitters still tuck babies in on their stomachs.

- When babies are awake, they should spend time on their stomachs so they can work on controlling their heads, pushing themselves up, and other feats of infant strength and coordination. This waking "tummy time" may also help prevent flat spots from developing on the back of your son's head. (Another way to prevent flattening is to make sure an infant's head is in different positions when he lies in the crib. If the baby usually turns his head to the right to see the doorway or a mobile, change his orientation so he has to look left to see it, or move the mobile. In any case, these flat spots are temporary and do no damage.)

- If your son can roll from his back to his stomach, but can't roll back, you should roll him back. Once he can roll from his stomach to his back, you can let him sleep in whatever position he assumes after you put him down on his back.

- The recommendation that babies sleep on their backs may not apply to some with certain medical conditions. Your health-care provider can advise you on which position is best for your son.

Physical Growth

Your son is growing by leaps and bounds every day (probably every minute!). He is gaining weight and growing in length at amazing speed. If he is feeding regularly without excessive vomiting or fussiness, he will grow as expected and right on track according to the standard growth charts.

GROWTH CHART

In Appendix A you'll find the growth charts your baby's doctor uses to keep track of his weight and length. You can plot your big boy's growth on these charts. Just keep in mind these are general averages and your son is unique. Always talk to your doctor about any growth concerns you have and use the charts only as a guide to compare your son with typical growth patterns.

Your Boy's Developing Senses: The parts of the brain that process information from the sense of touch are more developed at birth than those involved in vision or hearing. So it's touch that first gives your son a way to judge and react to his surroundings. Touch also gives him an emotional sense of security. In this way, it becomes an important component in the bonding process.

Although touching your son is unavoidable in day-to-day care, that's not the only kind of touch he needs. Take time to stroke his skin while bathing and diapering. Learn more about the art of baby massage as a way of improving your connection with your son. And keep in mind that each baby is unique in the way he processes stimulation. Some will immediately cuddle and coo and obviously enjoy being handled and stroked. Others will stiffen and arch their backs and show other signs of being a noncuddler. Experimentation and practice will help you find when and how you can touch your son in ways that will make you both feel comfortable and attached.

Emotional Development

Beyond feeding and diapering, our most important parenting job is to make our children feel loved. Giving our kids love enables them to value and love themselves. It teaches them how to love and relate to other people. And it allows them to become emotionally stable people. This strong emotional development begins at birth and continues throughout childhood through the process of bonding and attachment.

THE TRUTH ABOUT BONDING

Child psychologists tell us that it is very important to bond with our babies so they can develop strong emotional attachments to us and become secure and confident adults. I'm sure this is absolutely true, but I've always found the word *bonding* to be a bit misleading. It gives the impression of an epoxy glue–type union that, in a moment's time, adheres two beings together forever. Child psychologists tell us that's not really what bonding is all about. Human bonding is a gradual process that begins before a child's birth and continues throughout childhood.

Some believe there is a "critical" bonding period immediately after birth. This notion leaves many new parents feeling guilty and depressed when in the moments after childbirth they feel little more than exhaustion and a vague sense of fondness toward their newly arrived child. Quite commonly, truthful women admit, "I thought it would be love at first sight, but when I first looked at my son, 'love' was hardly my reaction." This idea of instant bonding is also quite upsetting to adoptive parents who are not available to the child immediately after birth. It's equally distressing to parents who are separated from their babies because either the baby or the mother needs prompt medical care.

Fortunately for parents who worry they've missed their chance to form a lasting attachment to their child, bonding does not happen in an instantaneous and magical moment. It happens each day in the routine interactions between a parent and a child—not in the perfunctory acts of feeding and changing diapers, but in the smiles, coos, and moments of eye contact that occur during these activities. It happens as parents learn about and respond to their baby's patterns, temperament, likes and dislikes, and unique daily rhythms. And it happens as babies become aware of their parents' smell, sound, and touch.

Bonding doesn't happen instantly, but it is very important that the process does occur. A secure parent/child relationship forms the basis for all later emotional attachments and it lays the groundwork that will enable children to seek and achieve loving and secure relationships as adults. Emotional attachment also contributes to the infant's overall mental and physical growth. Studies repeatedly find that babies who are deprived of the opportunity for emotional attachment are at risk for suffering the failure-to-thrive syndrome. This is a collection of symptoms that occur for no apparent physical reason. They include loss of weight, failure to grow, and a disruption in physical and mental development. When later cared for by emotionally involved and loving caretakers who provide an opportunity to form a loving relationship, infants resume normal mental and physical development.

Like any love relationship, bonding develops in gradual stages and improves and deepens with time and attention. To nurture that bonding process with your son, try these three simple ideas suggested in my book *Ages and Stages*:

☐ Consistently and immediately respond to your baby's cries of distress.

☐ Give much physical contact. Babies feel safer, sleep better, gain more weight, and are more interested in being with people when they are often cuddled, held, and stroked. The importance of loving touch cannot be overemphasized.

☐ Play with your son. Even in the first few months of life, infants enjoy games like peek-a-boo and songs. This creates a pleasure bond that encourages affection and attachment.

THE MYTH OF THE MAMA'S BOY

A very special bond often develops between dads and their sons. It's Dad who teaches junior how to fish or hit a ball. It's Dad who fixes toys when they break and patches up knees when they're scraped. But there's also a belief in some families that a dad shouldn't get too gushy or lovey with his boy; that it's the dad's job to rough him up and keep him tough. Sadly, this belief keeps some dads from ever really bonding with their baby boys, and it can make it difficult for the infant to attach positively and lovingly to his father.

For the last quarter of a century, Alice Sterling Honig, Ph.D., professor emerita of child and family studies in the College of Human Services and Health Professions at Syracuse University and a Fellow of the American Psychological Association and the Society for Research in Child Development, has studied the ways parents bond with their babies.

Dr. Honig believes that parents who hesitate to "baby" their infant son for fear that they will create a "sissy" or a "mama's boy" are missing the opportunity to get close and intimate with him. Acting critical or harshly toward baby boys may create a society of grown men who do not know how to form loving adult attachments. "Baby boys," she says adamantly, "are far more vulnerable and fragile than baby girls. They are much needier. They need to be protected and cuddled."

Some dads have a particularly hard time getting close to their sons. They're afraid that if they hold and caress a boy and are responsive to his cries, they will raise a spoiled, weak male who cries when he's physically or emotionally hurt. Some mistakenly believe that homosexual men were overly coddled as infants. This is a mistaken notion in our society that has a serious negative consequence for little boys, according to Dr. Honig. She remembers one case in her private practice when she was preparing to do intelligence testing with a twelve-month-old boy. She handed him a doll so he could point out the eyes, feet, and so on. But the boy drew back as if afraid of the little doll. "The mom explained, 'Oh, his dad won't let him touch a doll. He doesn't want his son to grow up to be a sissy or a homosexual.' This father thought that giving his son a security 'lovey' like a doll or a stuffed animal or a blanket that the child could cuddle up and sleep with would in some way weaken him as a male. This is exactly why some men grow up to be angry and violent. They are denied the opportunity for love and attachment when they're infants by fathers who think baby boys must be tough, and therefore deny them the tender loving care they need."

Your little boy needs the comfort of his dad's loving touch. Dr. Honig says research shows us that male infants need even more stroking, cuddling, and attention than baby girls. "Every time you change your baby boy's diaper," advises Dr. Honig, "stroke his tummy. Coo to him how gorgeous he is, how delicious he is, how much you love him. Kiss his toes, stroke his head. He will feel 'I am lovable! I am worthwhile!' That's a priceless message from a dad. That is what will make him a strong male."

Cognitive Development

Here's an interesting tidbit: Your son's brain grows and develops faster during this first year than at any other time in his life. You do not, however, need expensive or high-tech toys to encourage his intellectual growth at this early stage. Talking and singing to your son and playing games with his fingers and toes are fun and effective ways to boost brainpower.

EARLY LANGUAGE DEVELOPMENT

Some parents feel a little awkward talking to a little person who doesn't talk back. Although it's true that infants don't make the best conversationalists, they do enjoy and learn from conversational-type chatter. So, shake off that silly feeling and strike up a conversation with your son. Ask him questions. Pause for answers. Loosen up. Laugh. Joke. Enjoy. Don't make the mistake of shying away from baby talk. It's a wonderful way to entertain, educate, and love your son. And you'll probably never find such an eager listener ever again!

Here are a few simple guidelines to encourage early language development:

- Try to eliminate background noise like the TV or radio. It's difficult for an infant to concentrate on your voice when there are other sounds to listen to.

STAGES OF INFANT LANGUAGE DEVELOPMENT

As in most other areas of development, babies learn language at different rates and in varied ways. Some coo pleasantly; others grunt and squeak. Some babble incessantly; others listen intently. But along the way, you'll find these general signs of language growth:

Newborns	Listen to your voice. Vocalize by crying. Enjoy your singing and listening to music.
One to three-month-olds	Coo pleasantly. Make mostly vowel sounds. Will initiate communication, repeat sounds, and respond when given the opportunity.

- Use a higher than usual pitch in a singsong manner. Studies show that high-pitched sounds attract an infant's attention, and melodic intonation keeps that attention longer than normal adult conversational tone.

- Speak slowly and use simple words and short sentences. In casual conversation, many adults tend to slur words and ramble one sentence into the next. Speaking clearly and simply will help your baby become accustomed to the sounds of specific words and basic sentence structures.

- Engage your son's interest in conversation by keeping your face about twelve inches from his, using an animated style, and frequently changing your facial expressions.

■ When talking to your son, pause occasionally, as if waiting for a response. Ask questions and allow a few moments of silence to pass before continuing the conversation. These "conversations" teach lessons about tone, pacing, and taking turns when talking to someone else. As early as one month of age, you may be surprised to hear a cooing response.

GAMES BABY BOYS LOVE

Your newborn looks like he's ready for action as his arms and legs move, kick, and punch the air. But these motions are simply reflexes that he cannot consciously start or stop. Fine motor skills that will allow your son to grab hold of his toys to explore and play will develop not in an orderly progression, but at an uneven pace filled with rapid spurts and harmless delays. You can help your son develop the fine motor skills so important to his growth and development through infant games and play.

The hands of a newborn are closed most of the time and, like the rest of his body, he has little control over them. But in a wonderful innate reflex, if you touch his palm, he will unconsciously open his hand and clutch your finger. This reflex disappears within two to three months. During this time your baby will also grasp at any object placed in his hand, but without any awareness that he is doing so. Then, the fist will relax and he will drop the object, still unaware of what he has done. But it's all part of his developing abilities. By two weeks, he may begin flailing at objects that interest him, although he can't yet grasp them without your help. That's a good time to play with your son by showing him a brightly colored toy with strong, contrasting colors. Hold it just out of reach and watch him focus on it and begin to wave his arms and move his legs in excitement. Bring the object down to his hand and let him grab on. If you give him a baby rattle, for example, he will clutch it and shake it with vigor (although not with intentional will) and then suddenly drop it as his hand opens.

By eight weeks, although he still has not developed a deliberate grasp, your son will begin to discover and play with his hands. Using the sense of touch alone, he will explore his fingers and bring them to his mouth for further investigation. The mouth has many nerve endings, which makes it an ideal tool for learning.

At three months, he will add the sense of sight to his daily "play" and stare at his fingers in absolute awe. With fascination, he will watch them move and wiggle for long stretches of time. At this age, his own hands may be his favorite toy.

When hand-eye coordination begins to develop between the ages of two and four months, your son will discover the joy of focusing on an object and reaching out to intentionally grab it. Once in hand, it will go immediately to his mouth for further exploration.

Your newborn's escalating alertness allows for more time for active play as the weeks go on. Try a few different things to see what he enjoys and responds to. Show him rattles and demonstrate how they can make noise. Play with textured objects such as stuffed animals, guiding his hand to touch them. Gently tickle and kiss his tummy and feet. Hold a rattle or small toy in front of him and allow him to track it with his eyes.

By three months, your son will be ready for some good ol' baby games. This is when games that repeat a sequence of rhyming words are especially fun. In a singsongy voice, try "Pat-a-Cake," "Row Row Row Your Boat," and "Ring Around the Rosey."

MOM AND DAD PLAY STYLES

Right from infancy, moms and dads have different play styles. As researchers observed parents playing with their infants, they found that moms often contain a baby's movements by holding his legs or hips, while calming him down with a soft voice, slow speech, and repeated rhythmic phrases. Fathers, on the other hand, often poke their baby, pedal his legs, make loud, abrupt noises, and stimulate him to higher pitches of excitement.

It's important to respect your son's feelings about playtime. When he is hungry, tired, or uncomfortable, meet those needs first before attempting to play. And pace your games according to his reactions. Keep going only as long as he remains interested and stop when he seems to have had enough.

Social Development

Like all newborns, your baby boy certainly isn't a very good conversationalist, he doesn't mind his manners, and he has a limited social calendar. Still, he is a very social being. You can help him get to know his family and his world by providing him with early opportunities for social stimulation and separation experiences.

EARLY SOCIAL STIMULATION

Babies need to see, hear, and touch people to learn about their world and how they fit into it. So don't sequester your son in his quiet nursery. Make him a part of your family right from the beginning. Bring him into the kitchen to watch you cook and prepare meals. Let him join you at dinner and listen to your social conversations. Let him partake in social gatherings, holiday parties, and outdoor excursions.

Your son's temperament will largely determine the degree of social stimulation he's ready for. Your baby may love to be in the middle of things when he is awake, or you may notice that he wants only small doses of excitement at certain times of the day. To find just the right degree of social stimulation that's best for your son, take your cues from him!

When he is ready for social interaction by three months, he will meet your gaze and smile, following you with his eyes as you come and go. He will reach toward you. He will become more alert when you speak to him. He'll also carefully watch and make noises in response to other things that interest him, such as toys, his own reflection in the mirror, or friendly visitors.

New babies can also let you know when they've had enough attention. Crying is the most obvious cue, but they also will sneeze, pass gas, or yawn when they need to shut down for a while. Your son may also turn his face away from you. These signs of irritability when you're trying to play and be social are not a rejection of you. They are his attempts to communicate the best he can.

STEPS TOWARD SEPARATION

Your son may begin to show just how much he loves you—and only you—as early as three months. As he learns to distinguish himself from others, he may cry at the sight of unfamiliar faces, and he may reject people who look different than you—eyeglasses or a beard will send some babies into hysterics.

When this happened to my firstborn, I tried to keep him happy by staying at home with him. I turned down all baby-sitting offers even from my mother. If I had to leave him with a sitter, I would sneak out when he wasn't looking (or even awake). I learned the hard way that this strategy for avoiding heartbreaking good-bye scenes deprived my son of the opportunity to rehearse separation and set us both up for even worse episodes of separation anxiety between six and twelve months.

All mentally healthy children will go through a period of sepa-

THE SQUEAKY WHEEL

Babies who make a lot of noise and complain when they're left alone get the most social stimulation. They demand to be a part of the action at all times. On the other hand, quiet "good" babies, who are content to lie in their cribs alone often miss out on necessary social stimulation. Of course, it's tempting to let quiet babies lie, but your quiet son shouldn't miss out on social stimulation just because he's less demanding.

ration anxiety. But you can lessen the degree of upset by taking some preparatory steps while your son is still in infancy.

Once your son is one month old, create regular opportunities for separation. Call upon willing relatives, find a reliable sitter, or trade sitting time with another mother so you can leave him at least once a week for one- to two-hour periods. This will establish a comfortable routine for your son and will also give you time to schedule weekly dates with your partner, or do something else just for you. Starting this routine soon after birth has advantages because your baby won't yet protest being left behind, and setting up regular separation time will help both you and your son continue this schedule when he gets old enough to complain about your absence.

Separation "games" can help your son understand that when you leave, you also come back. When he is old enough to notice when you enter and leave a room, leave for a brief period of time, but maintain voice contact. Then return directly to him with a playful tickle or cuddle. Over time, leave the room for increasingly longer periods to teach him that just because you're out of sight, it doesn't mean you've disappeared. Peek-a-boo and hide-and-seek are also playful ways to teach the reassuring reality of object permanence.

If you find yourself feeling guilty or apprehensive at the thought of leaving your infant son, you can ease your own separation anxiety by following these guidelines:

Find a capable sitter. Family members are the most desirable sitters, but sometimes they are not available on a regular basis. Therefore, you may need to find a competent, caring person you can count on. The more confidence you have in your sitter, the less worried you'll feel while you're gone.

Never sneak out. It's easier and faster to duck out the door when your son isn't looking, but it defeats the goal of easing separation anxiety. It's confusing and upsetting, even to an infant, to suddenly realize that you're not around and have no idea where you are or if you'll be back. Let your baby see you depart and later see you come back. It won't take long before he learns that leaving is not forever.

Stay calm. Emotions are contagious. Parents who appear worried about separation pass this feeling on to their children. Don't prolong your good-byes by rushing back for another kiss. Don't spend too much time sharing your forlorn expression and sorrowful tone of voice. Say good-bye cheerfully and then leave.

Although you can't eliminate the separation anxiety stage from your son's developmental calendar, early separation experiences can ease the upset of this trying time. They can also teach babies a valuable lesson: When Mom and Dad leave, babies can trust other adults until they return—and they always do return.

Choosing Childcare

If you and your partner are going back to work shortly after the birth of your son, childcare is of course a top priority. Finding just the right type of care can take much effort, but when you make arrangements that you trust, the peace of mind you get in return is well worth the time spent making the right choice.

Here are some guidelines to help you select a child-care arrangement that will be best for both you and your baby.

SELECTING A CAREGIVER

There are several types of child-care arrangements to choose from. These include in-home care, home-based care, and day-care centers. I have used all three types at different times while raising my children and have found that they each have their good and bad points. So think about the pros and cons of each one before making your decision.

In-home care: In-home care allows your baby to stay in his own home with a sitter, which may be a family member, a nanny, or an au pair. This type of care gives you greater flexibility. You can accept overtime or attend late meetings and not worry about child-care arrangements. In-home care is also usually more personal and allows your son to stay at home without the jostling and inconvenience of being carried to and from another location in all sorts of weather. Another bonus is that your caregiver will likely watch your child even when he is sick, which is usually out of the question at day-care facilities.

There is a downside to in-home care. It's usually the most expensive option (unless you've hired a family member). Also, if your caregiver becomes ill and cannot watch your child, there's no backup. Finally, if you opt for a live-in nanny or au pair, you and your family may find you lose some privacy at home.

Home-based daycare: Home-based daycare provides care for a child in the caregiver's home, often with one adult supervising several children. The benefits of this type of care include a small group size (usually), a more home-like setting, and flexibility of hours.

On the other hand, home-based daycare is not as strictly regulated as day-care centers are, and the laws on licensing are different from state to state. Also, many of these caregivers are not formally trained, although they often have young children of their own. And, if the caregiver is ill, parents are left without backup arrangements for their children.

BABY-SITTER CHECKLIST

House facts:

House address: _____

House phone #: _____

Our cell phone #: _____

This is where you can reach us:

_____   _____   _____

Location   Address   Phone #

If we can't be reached, call:

Name: _____

Phone: _____

Phone numbers for emergency help:

Emergency: 911

Police: _____

Fire Department: _____

Poison Control: _____

Pediatrician: _____

Health Insurance Info:

Company: _____

Group #: _____

ID#: _____

Day-care center: Daycare in a center, preschool, nursery school, or provided by your workplace offers several advantages. It is more likely to be run in accordance with state regulations that set minimum standards for staff-child ratios, group size, staff training, and building safety. Additionally, day-care centers usually take children from six-week-old infants to school age. Caregivers usually have training in early childhood development, and a staff illness doesn't affect reliable care of your child.

The disadvantages of a daycare center include: There are often waiting lists because of a limited number of licensed centers, they usually have a more structured environment for your child because of the focus on regulations, they tend to have frequent turnover of staff, and usually offer inflexible pick-up and drop-off times.

CHILDCARE CRITERIA CHECKLIST

While considering the types of childcare, remember there are different guidelines depending on the age of your son. For infant care, finding a completely trustworthy caretaker is critical because your baby cannot tell you if he is subject to neglect or abusive behavior. If you're thinking about an out-of-home arrangement, visit the facility and look closely at these factors:

☐ Are all infants fed in the upright position, as they should be? Or are bottles propped up on pillows for feedings?

☐ Are all infants put to sleep lying on their backs?

☐ Are caretakers engaged with the children—not sitting around just watching them (or the TV)?

☐ Are children given lots of smiles and approval?

☐ Are infants separated from older children (who might accidentally hurt them)?

☐ Is there an open-door policy on visits from parents?

☐ Are sick children mingled in with the rest?

If you've opted to hire an in-home caregiver such as a nanny, be thorough:

☐ Interview the applicants at least twice.

☐ Ask for several references and check them all.

☐ If the caregiver will be driving your child, check his or her driving record.

☐ Outline all expected duties: hours, salary, paid vacation, and sick leave.

Whether home-based or center-based, slowly ease your baby into the new situation. Visit the center several times and leave your child for short periods (if allowed) before leaving him for the entire day. Or, invite your new nanny or au pair over for lunch. Let her care for your baby while you stay nearby to observe. Give your son a chance to get to know his or her voice and smell before you leave.

Leaving my babies behind in the care of another person was always very difficult. I'm not sure whether I worried about not being in control of my child's life, that something bad would happen

PLAN FOR EMERGENCIES

Be sure to give your caregiver all emergency contacts. Write down your work, beeper, and cell phone numbers, plus your e-mail addresses. Make sure the caregiver knows what to do in an emergency and provide contacts for friends, relatives, and your child's physician.

while I was gone, or that I secretly feared that my baby would love the caregiver more than me. It was probably a combination of all three. But looking back, I realize that these caregivers were an essential link that helped me balance the responsibilities of my job and family. Fortunately, my children have grown up to be happy, stable people—no worse for their days in childcare.

Moving Through Boyhood

As your son makes it through his third month of life, you can finally exhale. You'll both certainly be in one piece. You'll be better acquainted with each other. And you'll both be ready to move into the next stage of this wonderful time of boyhood—the four- to seven-month period when your newborn turns into a little social being full of giggles, smiles, and surprises.

MY BABY BOY

It is hard to choose baby clothes for my boy. For my daughter I worked so hard not to choose colors that are considered just for girls (although we received so many pink dresses as gifts anyway). But for my son I am more conscious not to choose colors that are considered just for girls. My daughter can wear any color, but I don't think some colors, like pink, are appropriate for my son.

—Melda N. Yildiz
Mother of a 6-year-old daughter and a 5-month-old son

Three

Settling In

Your Boy from Four to Seven Months

Months four through seven of your son's life will be filled with new adventures. You'll find he is becoming more aware of you and his own role in the world. He is now ready to "talk" to anyone willing to listen, to laugh at funny faces, and giggle with anticipation as you prepare his bath. This is a wonderful time to get to know the little person inside and smother him with love.

Feeding a Growing Appetite

Boy, could my Joey eat! I had planned to breast-feed him for the first year, but he was wearing me out. So at six months, I began to supplement his feedings with formula and offered him an occasional teaspoon of baby cereal. The American Academy of Pediatrics wouldn't agree with my decision (it says that most babies need only breast milk or formula for the first six months, or even longer if food allergies run in the family), but to calm hungry babies, many parents introduce solid foods between four and six months, when their baby seems ready to handle it.

Although your son isn't yet ready for a Big Mac, you might introduce some solid foods after talking to your doctor once you see these signs of readiness:

☐ He can sit alone or hold his head up when propped in a sitting position.

☐ He can turn his head to avoid something unpleasant.

☐ He shows interest in food. (He may try to grab your lunch or track each forkful with his eyes as it moves toward your lips.)

☐ He has lost the tongue-thrust reflex. (This reflex leads a newborn to push out foreign matter that enters his mouth. If your son still has it, you'll know it after a few tries at feeding because the food that goes in will come right back out. If that happens, you should wait a few weeks and try again.)

Okay, so you're little fella is ready for a solid meal! This is a big step, so take it slow. Your son's doctor will tell you that you shouldn't make an abrupt switch from bottle or breast milk to solid food. At first, continue to nurse or bottle-feed your son while you offer small amounts of solid food only once or twice a day. When babies first start eating solids, they will often eat only a teaspoon or two at a meal. Even after a month or two they may be taking in only three to four tablespoons a day of food, with the rest of their calories coming from breast milk or formula. Most doctors agree that until your child approaches his first birthday, solid food will supply some extra calories, but he should take most of his calories and nutrition from breast milk or formula.

FIRST FOODS

Doctors recommend that you introduce solid foods with small amounts of a single food, and offer only that food for several days. Then, you can add new foods one at a time, serving each one a few times before adding the next. This slow introduction will enable you to watch for possible bad reactions and allergies. If the baby gets a rash or diarrhea, for example, after eating one food for two days, it's easy to tell which food caused it. Once a food has been introduced for three to five days with no problem, you can move onto another.

Typically, the first food offered is a single-grain, iron-fortified baby cereal (usually rice cereal), followed by baby oatmeal or barley cereal. Baby cereals come ready-to-eat or as dry flakes, to be mixed with breast milk, formula, or water. (Don't mix them with cow's milk until your son is a year old.) If you get the ready-to-eat kind, you'll waste a lot of it because your son will eat just a little at first and you shouldn't keep the leftovers, even in the refrigerator, for more than a day or two. In either case, you should thin the cereal—in the beginning, it should have the consistency of thickened milk.

You can follow up the cereal with pureed fruit (such as banana, peach, apple, or pear, but not citrus fruit) or pureed vegetables (especially carrots, peas, squash, sweet potatoes, or green beans). Then you might start pureed meats or chicken. (Some babies seem to dislike meat until they are older; a vegetarian diet for infants is just fine.)

You might introduce finger foods when your baby has developed enough fine motor control to hold foods and bring them to his mouth, chew (or I should say *gum*), and swallow. This will probably happen sometime between six and seven months of age. Start out with small cereal pieces (like Cheerios) and let him explore the fun of feeding himself. Wait to introduce finger foods like fruit or hot dogs—right now his ability to chew is not firmly established and these foods pose a choking risk.

BABY FOOD: STORE-BOUGHT OR HOMEMADE?

I made all my own food for my first two babies. But by the time the third one came around, I was so busy that store-bought baby food suddenly looked just fine to me. All three of my children grew healthy and strong, and all three developed their own taste in later years for commercial, sweetened foods that I had hoped my first two would be spared. So choose whichever is best for your lifestyle regardless of what friends and family say.

Many parents find it's best to use both kinds—buying some baby food for convenience, especially for meals away from home, but making some other meals by pureeing or grinding regular food (as explained a bit later in this chapter). Do whatever makes mealtimes more pleasant for you and your son.

Commercial Baby Foods: Commercial baby food is convenient and consistent in taste and nutritional value. It's very safe, in terms of being canned without bacterial contamination, and doesn't need refrigeration unless jars have been opened. Like other processed foods, baby food tends to be lower in pesticide residues than some fresh produce. These days, most baby foods for the youngest children (labeled "Stage 1") are single foods without added salt, sugar, or fillers. Some baby foods even taste pretty good.

If you buy commercial baby food, follow these guidelines:

1. Read the labels. Baby food is formulated for babies of varying ages. Choose ones that match your child's age.

2. Avoid the baby-food desserts. Your son is better off without a lot of added sugar and without coming to expect a sweet finish to every meal.

3. Juices marketed for babies cost more, but most docs say they aren't necessary. You should be fine with any 100 percent juice that has been pasteurized.

4. When you open a jar of baby food for the first time, you should see the center of the lid pop up, as the airtight seal is broken. If it doesn't, don't use the jar.

Homemade Baby Food: If you prefer to make your own baby food, you'll find that it is less costly and usually tastier than commercial baby food. If you make it each day, your baby will get used to the livelier tastes of fresh vegetables and may learn quicker about the pleasures of healthy eating.

However, you should be careful about the fruits and vegetables you choose—and when possible, go organic. Regular produce does not have to meet the same standards as produce grown for baby food manufacturers. So if you're not careful, you may end up feeding your baby more pesticides than if you spooned food from the jar.

If you make your own baby food, follow these guidelines:

1. If you want to prepare more than one day's worth of food at a time, freeze the extra portions, rather than trying to can baby food yourself. (If you freeze pureed food in an ice-cube tray, you can easily pop out one cube at a time.)

2. Choose raw ingredients and peel or wash them thoroughly.

3. If you plan to puree or chop processed adult foods, such as canned fruit or frozen vegetables, read the labels to be sure they are not high in salt (sodium), sugar, or other ingredients you don't want to feed your baby. Canned soups and canned pasta with sauce, for example, often contain large amounts of salt.

BACTERIA ALERT

Whether you use commercial baby food or make your own, place the amount of food you want to use at one feeding in a bowl or food tray and put the rest in the refrigerator in a container with a tight seal. Any food that is not used from that feeding should be thrown away. *Do not refrigerate the leftovers.* A baby's saliva introduces bacteria into the food, so you should not use it again at another feeding.

4.   You can use a blender, food processor, or food mill to chop up food to the proper consistency for babies. Many parents swear by small, plastic food mills that are portable for grinding on the go.

HOW TO FEED YOUR SON

It seems that the logical advice here would be: Put food on a spoon and place the spoon in your child's mouth. But like so many new adventures with your son, it's usually not that easy. It took a three-ring circus to get food into my Joey because if he wasn't distracted, he made it impossible to get the spoon to his mouth before he grabbed it. I finally figured out a way to hold him and his arms during feeding times. I held him upright close to my body in my left arm. I put his right arm behind my body and I held down his other arm with my left hand. Now I could use my right hand to feed him. Perhaps a straightjacket would have been easier, but this worked just fine for us!

We all have to find the best method, but here are some tips that might make it easier for you. In the beginning, nurse or bottle-feed your baby a little bit before putting him in the seat so he is not overly hungry. Show him the food and let him touch it, even smear it around if he wants to. Then take a small infant spoon (the rubber-coated kind are gentle in the mouth), a demitasse spoon, or a half-teaspoon from a measuring-spoon set. Put a tiny bit of food on the spoon and place the spoon between his lips. Do not put it far back on his tongue or he may gag.

Once your son tastes the food, he may suck it off the spoon and open his mouth for more. He may spit it out but seem interested.

FOODS TO AVOID

Some foods are more likely than others to cause allergic or other adverse reactions in babies. Chief among these foods are cow's milk, eggs, soy, peanuts, and wheat, as well as citrus fruits (including orange juice), shellfish, other nuts, and corn. It is best not to give these to your son until he is eating the foods mentioned earlier. If food allergies run in your family, talk to your doctor before feeding him these foods. Delaying them may reduce the chance of developing allergies. Here are tips on some potential problem foods:

- **Cow's milk.** Because its concentrations of protein and minerals are too high for young infants, cow's milk should not be given until a baby is one year old. Even after that age, if you have stopped breast-feeding, your child may be better off drinking iron-fortified formula, rather than cow's milk, especially if he is not eating enough iron-rich food, such as meat or iron-fortified cereal. Contrary to what many people think, cow's milk is not essential for babies as long as they get enough calcium and protein from other sources. Cheese and yogurt are good sources of both. Talk to your son's doctor about this. By age five, some children—especially those of African, Asian, or Native American descent—may start to have trouble digesting lactose, a milk sugar. Special milk and pills can help with this lactose intolerance, which continues into adulthood.

- **Peanuts and peanut butter.** These products can pose a double risk—as a possible cause of allergies and as a choking hazard. (Toddlers and babies can choke on sticky globs of peanut butter as well as on the nuts themselves.) To be safe on both counts, wait until age three before giving peanut butter and then spread it on bread or crackers, rather than serving it plain. Wait until age four to serve nuts.

• **Honey and corn syrup.** Do not give these sweeteners to children who are less than one year old. They may contain bacterial spores that can cause botulism (a serious illness) in babies, but not in older children or adults.

He may gag, cry, or become upset. He may reach for the spoon himself. (Let him play with it. After a while, you can try to guide it to his mouth, or you can feed him with another spoon while he hangs onto the first.) As long as he seems interested, you can keep trying. Talk to your son in a pleasant tone throughout this process, explaining what you are doing.

Once he has had a few spoonfuls or seems tired of the process, finish up the feeding by offering more breast milk or formula. In the beginning, very little food will actually be swallowed, but never mind: The goal in the beginning is to teach him to eat, not to meet his nutritional needs with solid food.

A NOTE ON NEATNESS

Learning to eat can be a messy process—and likely to get much messier as your son gets older and starts feeding himself. For the next few years, much of his meal may end up on the floor. You can try to save yourself clean-up time by putting a small plastic drop cloth under his chair, but then you have to clean the plastic. Instead, put old newspaper under the chair that you can throw out afterward, or put down a cloth tablecloth that you can shake out and throw in the washing machine.

Bibs are a must! They come in all shapes and sizes. Whatever style you choose, use one at every meal to save yourself the trouble of having to give your son a complete change of clothes after eating. Plastic bibs are nice because they can be sponged off. The rigid plastic kind—which look a bit like a knight's breast plate—have a pocket at the bottom that catches dropped morsels. Be sure to take the bib off your son in between meals to avoid the risk of choking or strangulation, and be particularly careful with bibs that tie on with strings.

BABY BOYS: "IRON MEN" NEED MORE IRON

During and after my pregnancies, my doctor recommended that I take iron supplements to avoid iron deficiency anemia and the fatigue that it brings. As my babies grew (and fatigue became my new best friend), I switched to a multivitamin that contained iron in the hope that the extra dosage could somehow boost me through the long, hectic days. During this time, my sons took their daily vitamin drops, though it never occurred to me that they might need additional iron—more so than their little sister. But that's the finding of a very recent study. Indeed, the need is greatest in breast-fed baby boys.

The authors of this study, published in *Pediatrics* magazine, randomly placed 263 full-term, breast-fed infants into two groups at four months of age: one group received iron supplements, the other a placebo. When blood samples were taken at four, six, and nine months of age, each testing found that the boys had significantly lower iron levels. At nine months, boys had a ten-fold higher risk of having iron deficiency anemia than the girls. This finding remained significant even in the group taking the iron supplementation.

The researchers concluded that there are substantial sex differences in the levels of hemoglobin and other indicators of iron status during infancy. They felt that some of these differences may be genetically determined, but others appeared to reflect an increased incidence of true iron deficiency in boys.

Your son's doctor may not know of this finding or may not agree. But it's worth mentioning and perhaps asking for a blood test for iron deficiency at your baby's next visit.

Dressing Baby Boys

I've often suspected that we buy blue "boy" clothing for our little sons because that's all we can find in the stores. We don't really have a choice about continuing the "pink is for girls and blue is for boys" mind-set if clothing designers offer no options. Right?

Well, not exactly, according to Freddie Curtis, director of fashion design and fashion merchandising programs at Harcum College in Bryn Mawr, Pennsylvania. Curtis knows what fashions sell for little boys and what don't. She makes baby blankets and sweaters that are sold in upscale boutiques in large metropolitan areas such as Philadelphia, Washington, D.C., New York City, Florida, and Houston. Curtis has found that it doesn't matter how sophisticated or educated parents may be, they still want to dress their baby boys in blue. "I'd like to offer a wider variety of colors," she says, "but people are very traditional, and they want blue for boys."

In the ten years Curtis has been selling children's fashions, she has seen no change in this preference. "Over all these years," she says, "the favorite color in my quilts for boys has been blue or navy check or navy-and-red plaid. Once in a while, I can sell pastel plaids in pale blue on white. This just never changes."

The stereotypes of color and fashion seem to be stronger for boys than girls. "Parents are more likely to accept girls dressing 'like boys,'" Curtis says, "than they are of having their sons dress 'like girls.' We don't mind dressing our girls in blue clothing or dungarees. But most parents don't like to see their sons wearing pink."

So, when you go out shopping for little-boy clothes and find they seem to only come in powder blue, navy blue, aqua blue, wedgewood blue, periwinkle blue, and so on, now you know why.

Grandparents, Trucks, and Footballs

Having loving grandparents is a blessing for all children. The importance of this relationship is supported by reams of research showing that children with the support of loving grandparents have a greater sense of family and of self-worth. I have always believed that there can never be too many loving adults in a child's life. But sometimes it's hard to remember this.

I raised my eldest son, Matt, in what I believed was the "right" way. We did not have a TV in the house. I made my own baby food from natural, organic products. I dressed him in gender-neutral colors and surrounded him with both "boy" and "girl" toys to avoid creating stereotypical attitudes. These things were important to me—but not to my mother.

When Grandma got the chance to spend a few hours alone with her grandson, she would nod and smile as I gave her my list of dos and don'ts, and then thoroughly enjoy spoiling him by breaking every rule I set. I would return to find my infant son plopped in front of her TV with a cowboy hat on his little head, smacking his lips over the jarred peach-apple cobbler baby food he'd just enjoyed. There were many fights over this difference of opinion about child-rearing—that I now regret.

My mom died before my other two children were born and before I grew to realize that the love she gave my son was far more important and valuable than the fact that the way she chose to give it was different than my own. But my mother-in-law stepped right up to continue the grandparental duty of spoiling her grandchildren in her own way. She gave me lots of opportunities over the years to learn how to compromise and balance her parenting style with my own.

One area that often needs rather heavy-handed balancing is the issue of gender stereotypes in toys and clothing. Thanks to the feminist movement in the 1970s, today's grandparents are far more aware of unnecessary gender stereotypes than in generations past. But when it comes to their own grandchildren, you may find that your parents and in-laws have some biased views that differ from your own.

Maureen O'Brien, Ph.D., director of parenting and child development at The First Years, Inc., in Avon Massachusetts, and author of *Watch Me Grow: I'm One-Two-Three,* says that from birth to age two a baby is learning who he is as a person and what it means to be a boy. As a developmental psychologist, she points out that any adult who spends a good amount of time with the baby will influence that development.

"Your son's grandparents come into the picture with a whole set of expectations: what they think babies should be like, what kind of activities they should be involved in, what kind of personality is 'appropriate' for the gender of the baby," O'Brien says. "They might also bring their own dashed expectations from when they were parents. Maybe they wanted a son but had only girls. Maybe they wanted a son who would excel in athletics, but got one who liked chess. Like parents, grandparents bring a whole lifetime of experience to their relationship with your son. This can be wonderful if those expectations are in line with what you want your child to be exposed to, but it can be quite a challenge if you don't agree."

O'Brien feels that your child's infancy is a good time to hash out this difference of opinion because your baby isn't yet aware of the push-pull that may go on between you and your own parents. By toddlerhood he'll be conscious of any differences you have. This is the time to explain yourself if you have strong feelings about the kinds of toys and clothing that grandparents should give to your child, or the kinds of play activities that are or aren't appropriate.

For example, some parents feel strongly that fairy tales are sexist and stereotypical. Your son won't notice this yet, but if these are the kind of stories he hears from infancy on, by the time he is three or four years old he will pick up the stereotypes and will act out the part. Your son will see himself as the hero, the conqueror, the savior. He will see girls as the helpless damsels in distress. When grandparents insist on reading and rereading these tales to their babies, a battle often erupts. The fight may be worthy, but O'Brien believes it's probably a losing one.

"If you want to bring up your child in a gender-neutral world," she says, "the reality is you don't have a chance because the world is not gender-neutral. You have to be realistic and realize that there is a whole world of influence that will show your children gender stereotypes." In fact, O'Brien says that by themselves these stereotypes are not necessarily a bad thing. In their neutral form, they are just one other way to categorize things. When kids are first starting to learn about the world, they do that in many ways: big things, little things; loud things, quiet things; girl things, boy things. It is a helpful way for them to put order in their world. Labeling is natural and harmless. It's when a category becomes biased that it can become troublesome: Girls are dainty and therefore helpless; boys are brave and therefore never cry. We contribute to this kind of gender bias when we scold our little boys for trying on Mommy's shoes or tell our daughters that they can't help Daddy with the yard work because girls shouldn't get dirty.

So if your son's grandparents are stuck on gender stereotypes and buy him only rough-and-tough toys, blue clothing, and he-man books, they're not going to create a problem that isn't already in the world at large, and which will eventually touch your child anyway.

Dr. O'Brien saw this in her own family. "I gave my baby boys plenty of dolls," she says, "but as they grew into the grade school years, they tossed them aside and spent more time with trucks. I can't blame myself or anyone else for that. But now that they're ten years old, I do notice that they have less stereotypical ideas than boys of my generation. When I talk about a doctor, for example, they will ask, "Is it a boy or a girl doctor?" The fact that they can ask that question shows me that my efforts have given them some degree of gender respect, and that after all was my goal."

If Grandma and Grandpa have stereotypical ideas and argue that you should throw your son's doll away and buy him a truck, you don't have to let this difference of opinion escalate into a major battle. When they arrive with one more truck or football, just say thanks with a smile and add it to the pile. When the grandparents leave, you can offer your son a balanced experience by giving him gender-neutral toys.

You'll find as your son grows that he will be exposed to many things that you don't like but can't control. Your goal in all these

SCIENCE SAYS

Although mothers talk to and hold sons more often in the first few weeks of life (possibly because boys tend to be more fussy after birth), the pattern reverses after two or three months. These studies found that throughout infancy, mothers are more warm and expressive with their daughters than with their sons, particularly when a male infant becomes a bit fussy or seems to resist her affection by looking away or crying. When this happens mothers interpret these signals differently according to gender. With a girl, they step up their efforts to comfort and soothe. With a boy, they back away and give the baby time to work out his discomfort by himself. The researchers feel that this response shows that even in the first few months of life, girls are subtly being encouraged to be sociable and responsive to others, while boys are allowed to be independent.

situations should be to make your home the place where he learns that he is valued and loved as a person regardless of the toys he plays with or the style of clothes he wears.

Sleep Tight

We all have a biological clock that governs our sleep-wake cycles, making us sleepy at certain times and wakeful at others. Our sleep-wake clock is "set" each day by darkness and light, especially exposure to bright morning light. Newborns do not have this biological rhythm and will wake and sleep around the clock regardless of daylight or nightfall. Then, usually by three months of age, they develop an internal sleep-wake clock.

You can help your son set his internal clock to better match your own simply by putting him to bed and waking him at the same time every day. A consistent waking time seems to be especially important to setting this clock and forming good sleep patterns.

Some babies develop regular sleep-wake patterns as early as six or eight weeks, but usually these patterns emerge around three or four months. At that age, most babies average three to five hours of sleep during the day, usually grouped into two or three naps, and ten to twelve hours at night, usually with an interruption or two for feeding.

I remember reading that most babies at this age sleep through the night—boy, did I feel that all three of my children had let me down—until I learned what the phrase *sleep through the night* really means. It is defined as sleeping five hours in a row. So if I put my babies down at 9 P.M. and they were up again at 2 A.M., they had slept "through the night" and I didn't even know it! With this in mind, it's probably best to put your son down as close to midnight as possible.

TEACHING YOUR SON TO FALL ASLEEP

If may seem unnecessary to teach a baby how to fall asleep—most do a pretty good job of that without any lessons. But if your son is six months old and still calling for you in the middle of the night, he needs to learn how to fall asleep *by himself*. If you always rock, feed, or soothe him to sleep, you take away his natural ability to self-soothe and therefore cause him to be more dependent on you.

I was the world's worst offender in this department. I had unknowingly taught my son Joey to connect my presence with falling asleep. Then, if I was not able (or willing) to always rock or feed him back to sleep, he would cry through the night (scream is closer to the truth). My middle son was two years old before he finally slept from nighttime to daybreak. That blessed event happened only after I took him to a crying baby clinic I saw advertised in the newspaper. I was at my wits' end and would do anything to make this child sleep by himself.

At the clinic I met Charles Schaefer, Ph.D., who offered me a plan. His method actually worked, and eventually I helped him write the book *Teach Your Baby to Sleep Through the Night*. Here are the basics:

1. **Say good night.** When you put your son to bed for the night, say good night and leave the bedroom *before* your child is asleep. Keep reminding yourself that your baby is capable of falling asleep on his own without your help. You just have to teach him how.

The bedroom should be exactly the same when you first say good night as it will be when your son wakes up in the middle of the night: no overhead light, no music, no parent.

2. Wait. If your son cries when you leave at bedtime or awakens crying at night, wait five minutes before responding.

3. Check. Then go and make a quick check on him to reassure yourself that he is all right. This quick check should be just that—quick. Stay with him only one or two minutes to clean up any mess or to make sure he is not feverish, in pain, too hot, or too cold. Do not pick him up. Rather:

☐ Go up close to him.

☐ Establish eye contact.

☐ Maintain a stern facial expression.

☐ Use a firm voice to say his name and give a simple, direct command such as, "Go to sleep."

☐ Do not scream, become hostile, or hit him.

☐ Do not sympathize, hug, or show your own distress.

4. Check again. If the crying persists for another twenty minutes after the first check, go again to check on your child and remind him that you expect sleep, not crying at this hour. Do not feed, rock, or pick him up. Leave again before he is asleep.

Repeat this procedure of briefly checking on your son after

every twenty-minute crying spell for as long as it takes him to finally get tired and fall asleep. If your child is crying softly or whimpering at the end of a twenty-minute period, do not go and check because he is probably close to falling asleep on his own.

Twenty minutes seems to be an optimal length of time to let infant night wakers cry. On many occasions they will fall back to sleep on their own after ten to fifteen minutes.

5. Stick to the daily schedule. Awaken your son at his usual wake time in the morning. Do not allow him to sleep any later regardless of how little sleep you or he had the night before. Also, keep his daily nap schedule intact. Do not allow him to take more or longer naps during the day. As tempting as it will be to make up for lost sleep during the day, try to resist. Doing so will disturb the wake-sleep rhythms you're trying to develop to ensure a good night's sleep.

Dr. Schaefer expected that this routine would teach my son to put himself to sleep in three nights. It took a grueling five, but it was worth it! My husband was sure through the whole ordeal that it would never work. He sometimes insisted that we bring our little screamer into our bed and forget the whole thing. But I was determined and refused to give in. I knew that the alternative was continued nights of disrupted sleep, rocking, walking, or sitting by his side until he fell asleep. I had had two years of being sleep deprived, exhausted, and irritable. It was time to do something about it. Besides (I kept reminding myself) Dr. Schaefer said that learning to calm himself can be a step in a child's long path to independence, fostering a sense of competence and self-confidence. As long it occurs in the context of a close, loving relationship, it causes no emotional damage.

Finally, this method was effective. In fact, it worked so well with my son, that when my daughter arrived three years later, my husband the skeptic was happy to try it as soon as she was six months old. Again, it worked (much more easily and quickly) and we saved ourselves the years of sleepless nights we had endured with our son.

If after trying this method for one week (without giving in occasionally!), your six-month-old continues to wake up several times each night and cry for your attention, talk to your pediatrician about it. There may be something else bothering him.

Childproofing Your Home

People without young children must have thought I had the worst sense of interior design on the planet. When my children were babies, my house looked like I had just moved in and hadn't yet put out the knickknacks, plants, and other decorative touches that make a house a home. But I learned very quickly that it was far better for all of us if breakables were packed away, sharp objects were moved to higher ground, and cabinets and drawers were locked tight.

I also learned that it's never "too soon" to start childproofing. While your son is between four and seven months, take a good look around your home and begin to think about safety. Because you can't predict the day he'll learn to roll over to the electrical cord, or scoot on his behind to the edge of the stairs, or eventually crawl across the room to the hot stove, take time now to prevent accidents and injuries by making a few simple changes in your household. Here's a list to get you started:

- Survey your house for hazards, then search again. Walk slowly through the house looking for potential danger. Then, crawl through the house to get a baby's perspective.

- Move all sharp objects, including knives, forks, vegetable peelers, and sewing or hobby implements out of reach or get latches and locks for their drawers and cabinets. Drawer latches of various designs are widely available through stores, catalogs, and websites that sell baby products.

- Move anything that could be swallowed into high or locked cabinets or closets. This includes medicines, vitamins, cleansers, cosmetics, detergents, stain removers, air fresheners, candles, and pet food. Regular human food can also choke a baby and should not be easy to get at.

- If you have drawers that can be pulled out all the way without stopping, install latches or stops so your son doesn't pull them out onto himself.

- Put outlet covers on or plugs in unused electric sockets.

- Check for hanging wires, blind cords, or the like that could be pulled down or could choke a baby.

- Move objects that could break or fall.

- Move high-risk furniture or make it safe. Tall bookcases and dressers should be secured to the walls with brackets, so that if your son climbs on them they won't tumble over on top of him. You can buy elasticized padding to put around the hard edges of tables that might be in a toddler's path.

■ Be prepared to install gates to block off staircases. (Use the kind that mounts to the wall with hardware.)

You won't catch all potential hazards (and so you should never leave your son "loose" and unsupervised). But this list should prevent the most obvious dangers. You should repeat this process every time your baby moves up in mobility—when he starts to crawl, walk, run, and climb.

CHECK FOR LEAD PAINT

Lead paint was banned in 1978 because it was found to cause lead poisoning. But if your home was built before that date, you should have painted areas, both exterior and interior, checked by the local department of health to see if your son is in danger of lead paint exposure.

Lead paint is seductively sweet. If young children eat paint chips or inhale lead dust, they can suffer lead poisoning. Milder forms of lead poisoning have been associated with learning problems, and severe cases can cause mental retardation and many physical problems. If lead paint is found in your home, ideally it should be removed or covered with paneling or plasterboard before the baby arrives. (Lead paint is best removed by professionals who know how to contain the lead dust it produces.) It is also important to identify areas coated with lead

FIVE SAFETY ITEMS
YOUR HOME SHOULD HAVE

To safeguard your baby in times of emergency, stock up on these five safety items:

☐ Smoke detectors

☐ Fire extinguishers

☐ Carbon monoxide detector

☐ Flashlights

☐ Escape ladder

paint if you plan to renovate rooms because such work can create and spread lead dust.

If you are a renter and your landlord refuses to have your apartment checked for lead, contact your local health department. Rules about if and when landlords can be required to remove or cover over lead paint vary from place to place. If your landlord resists following the rules, you may need to seek help from the health department, tenants' groups, or health advocacy groups.

Medical Care

The four- to seven-month old baby boy is a medical marvel. The healthy infant kicks, rocks, and rolls with vigor and gusto during all waking hours. But when he's not feeling well, he can't tell you about it, so you'll have to let any change in feeding and activity level tip you off. Sometimes you can handle the problem yourself; other times you'll need to call your son's doctor. The information in this section will help you decide which are normal childhood discomforts (like teething and overheating) and which need a professional's care.

ROUTINE AT-HOME HEALTH CARE

Every day you work hard to keep your little boy comfortable and happy. You change his diaper before his bottom gets red; you feed his tummy before he screams from hunger pains; you rock him, sing to him, and hold him close. Here are some pointers about keeping that comfort level high as the seasons change and as the pain of teething begins.

Seasonal care: Fresh air and a change of surroundings are good for you and your son, so take him out for walks in nice weather. But be careful to dress him properly—not too much and not too little.

An infant's body loses heat more readily than an older child or adult. This makes it difficult for his body to regulate temperature when he's exposed to excessive heat or cold during the first year or so of life. In general he should wear one more layer (of clothing or a blanket) than you do when it is cold.

If it is uncomfortably cold, keep him inside if possible. If you have to go out, dress him in warm sweaters or bunting bags over his other clothes and use a warm hat over his head and ears. You can shield his face from the cold with a blanket when he's outside, but hold it far enough from his nose and mouth so he can breathe easily.

To check whether your son is clothed warmly enough, feel his hands and feet and the skin on his chest. His hands and feet should be slightly cooler than his body but not cold. His chest should feel warm. If his hands, feet, and chest feel cold, take him into a warm room, unwrap him, and hold him close so the heat from your body warms him.

In warm or hot weather, you can ease up on the layers. Dress your son as you dress yourself to feel comfortable, while protecting him from direct sun rays.

Babies less than six months old should be kept out of direct sun entirely because they are prone to sunburn and heatstroke, both of which can be dangerous at this age. Keep your baby in the shade of a tree, umbrella, or stroller canopy. For years, the American Academy of Pediatrics recommended against putting sunblock on babies under six months because of concerns about the way their skin might absorb the chemicals. But in 1999, the Academy changed its position, saying that if clothing and shade to block the sun are not available, it may be reasonable to apply sunscreen to small areas, such as the face and back of the hands. Still, the best way to protect your child from the sun's ultraviolet rays is to keep him out of the sun altogether.

Teething: Although it's not time to bring on the steak, your son will probably cut his first teeth during this infant period. By the time babies are born, they have a full set of primary teeth (commonly called baby teeth) hidden below the gum line, as well as the beginnings of the permanent teeth that will come later. The first

TEETHING TIMELINE

Five to six months: Teething begins. The first tooth to appear is usually one in the bottom front. Because teeth appear in pairs, the second tooth (the mate to the lower incisor) will appear often within days of the first.

About eight months: The two upper front teeth will emerge.

By twelve months: The four incisors (on each side of the front teeth) appear and the first molars begin to emerge.

All twenty primary teeth—ten on top, ten on the bottom—are usually in by age three.

baby tooth usually breaks through when the baby is between four and seven months, although the big event may occur as early as three months or as late as twelve months.

Your son will let you know when he's teething. There's no mistaking the drool that will run down his chin all day long. He is also likely to chew on anything he gets his hands on to ease the discomfort. Some babies have short bursts of irritability, while others may seem cranky for weeks, crying frequently, waking more often and eating fretfully. Sometimes the process seems to be almost completely painless. As the gums grow tender and swollen, the body temperature may be a little higher than normal. But as a rule, teething does not cause high fever, diarrhea, earaches, runny noses or coughing (as your mother may have told you).

To make teething more pleasant for your son try these simple teething strategies:

- Wipe your son's face often with a soft cloth to remove the drool and prevent rashes or irritation.

- Place a clean flat cloth (such as a diaper not used for diapering) under his head when you lay him down to sleep. If he drools, you can replace it with a dry cloth without having to change the whole sheet.

- Try rubbing your son's gums with a clean finger. (Do not coat your finger with sugar or honey.)

- Give your son something firm to chew on, but be sure it's not small enough to swallow and can't break into pieces that might pose a choking risk. (Bagels, which are used as teething rings by some parents, are not a good choice for this reason. Neither are teething biscuits, despite their name, or frozen bananas.) Hard rubber teething rings can be good; look for one-piece models.

- Make it cold. Many babies seem to enjoy teething on objects that have been chilled but aren't rock-hard. Try freezing a clean wet washcloth for thirty minutes, then let your son chew on it. Or try a cool spoon.

- If your son seems to be in a lot of pain, it may be worth giving him acetaminophen drops, but consult his doctor first. Ditto for painkillers that are applied to the gums (such as Baby Orajel or Baby Anbesol). These provide relief for a short time, and may be just long enough to allow him to fall asleep.

- Never use old–home remedies such as placing an aspirin against the gum or rubbing the gum with any type of alcohol. And don't clean those little teeth with a fluoride tooth-paste. He may swallow some paste, which can result in tooth staining or surface irregularities on the enamel.

ROUTINE MEDICAL CHECKUP

Lots of us adults do not arrange for periodic routine medical checkups for ourselves, as we should. We put them off and plan to keep the appointment next year—usually with no major harm done. But when it comes to our babies, there's no putting it off. Infants need regular checkups on a rather strict schedule so that doctors can monitor their medical and developmental progress, give required inoculations, and catch any problems early on.

I never missed an infant checkup with my kids, but I can't say that I really knew why they were so important. So I've again asked Stephen Muething, M.D., section director of clinical services at Cincinnati Children's Hospital Medical Center, to tell us what happens at these checkups that he says most physicians will schedule for your son at four and six months of age.

Dr. Muething says that the physician will give your son a thorough physical as she did in previous visits. Again she will weigh and measure the baby, and then measure his head (a baby's head will grow about one-half inch every month for the first six months). She will listen to your son's heart and lungs with a stethoscope. She will examine his legs, feet, and overall skin color and condition, as well as the genitals. And finally, she will look at his eyes, nose, ears, and throat for signs of good health.

Your son will probably be given immunizations at one or both of these visits. The typical infant gets twelve immunization shots

within the first six months. This is far more than your parents remember. These shots protect children against: hepatitis B, polio,
measles, mumps, rubella (German measles), pertussis (whooping
cough), diphtheria, tetanus (lockjaw), Haemophilus influenzae type
b, pneumococcal infections, and chickenpox. Be sure to follow your
doctor's instructions on when these inoculations are due. The recommended schedule does change from time to time, but you can find
the most up-to-date recommended immunization schedule on the
website of the American Academy of Pediatrics at www.aap.org, or
the Centers For Disease Control at www.cdc.gov/nip/acip.

The four- and six-month visits are also the time when your
baby's doctor will want to hear about your son's feeding schedules.
Many moms who started nursing will now be adding some formula
or switching to formula entirely. And during this period, many
parents introduce some kind of solid foods. The doctor will discuss
your son's feedings and offer some advice on how to continue to
introduce new foods and watch for possible bad reactions.

Sleep is another subject that often concerns parents when babies
are between four and seven months old. "Some parents come in,"
says Dr. Muething, "with that look of fatigue, and I know that
sleep is an issue we need to talk about." If your son is not yet sleeping through the night, now is the time to talk about that.

After the basics are covered, Dr. Muething notes that parents
should be prepared to ask any questions they have. "After the first
few visits where parents are concerned about the baby's physical
health," he says, "they now start to focus on the baby's development. They want to make sure the baby is doing what he's supposed to be doing at the right time. Is he developing physically

and intellectually as he should be? Most often moms know something is wrong before the doctor says anything. They know it in their heart, but don't want to say it." These routine checkups give you an opportunity to make sure your baby is progressing as he should.

- At four to six months old, your infant should be able to sit with some support. And, he may also be able to roll over from his back to his side and from stomach to back.

- Your son should now have some hand-eye coordination and be able to grab at things he sees. He grabs at objects and brings his hands or the objects close to his face to his mouth. He also opens and closes his hands so that he can pick up and look at objects.

- All babies this age should be becoming social, track visually, interact with parents, smile responsively, coo, and make noise.

IT'S ALL IN THE BRAIN

The parietal lobe of the brain interprets sensations such as touch, pain, and temperature. The male brain in infants seems to block out some of sensory input, making boys less sensitive to physical sensations on the skin.

WHEN TO CALL THE DOCTOR

Whether or not to phone the doctor when your son is sick is a tough call. Here are some facts to help you answer the question "Should I?" or "Shouldn't I?":

If your son has symptoms of a cold, fever, or flu, you may wonder whether you should call the doctor. Dr. Meuthing says, "The way the baby is feeding is important when deciding whether or not to call the doctor. If the baby is feeding well, then we're not that concerned. But if he is not feeding well, or has stopped feeding completely, we want the parents to call. A baby's number one job is to eat and grow. If he can't get the job done, something is wrong, and we should check it out."

When you call the doctor because your son seems ill, it helps to be specific and focused, especially if you are not calling during office hours.

- Remind the doctor of your child's age, past and continuing medical problems (including low birth weight or prematurity), and any medications, including over-the-counter drugs or supplements, that he is taking.

- Describe the symptoms that led you to call. Say when the symptoms started, how they have changed, and how you have handled them so far. Be as specific as possible: Saying, "He usually wakes up to eat every four hours, but we've had to wake him for the last three feedings," is a description that tells the doctor more than if you just say the baby is unusually sleepy.

- Spell out what you are concerned about: "His cough seems to be getting worse, and now that it's bedtime I'm worried he'll have trouble breathing during the night."

- Mention all the symptoms that concern you, but don't mix in routine issues that could be dealt with some other time, such as whether to use a pacifier or start solid food.

- Take your son's temperature before you call and write it down, along with the time it was taken.

- If your son has vomited or has diarrhea, be prepared to describe when, how often, and what it looked like.

- Try to notice whether your son is urinating as much as usual. If not, be sure to tell the doctor.

- Have a pad at hand to write down instructions. Have your son's health record available to update and give additional information if necessary.

- Have the name and number of your pharmacy available in case the doctor wants to call in a prescription.

COMMON HEALTH CONCERNS

As your son spends less time in your protective arms and more time on the floor exploring his world, there's more to think about to keep him safe and healthy. A good childproofing plan as explained earlier should protect him from most harmful situations, but babies have a way of finding trouble even in the most guarded homes. Here are some tips you should keep in mind as your son reaches out to examine his world.

HOW TO HANDLE A CHOKING BABY

As your son begins to get around by rolling and scooting across the floor, he's bound to find interesting things to put in his mouth. A dropped coin or a forgotten watch battery is irresistible to your little explorer. But these are also choking hazards that can prevent airflow in and out of the lungs.

If the airway becomes blocked, your son will not be able to breathe or make normal sounds and his face will turn from bright red to blue. This situation calls for immediate intervention. If the situation appears critical, have someone call 911 while you determine the best course based on the following information.

Choking, coughing, but able to breathe: If your son is coughing but is still able to breathe and make noises, the airway is not fully blocked, and he will likely clear the airway by himself by coughing it up. Don't attempt to remove an object by trying to reach in and grasp it with your fingers. That could push it farther into the throat and totally block the airway. Instead, let the child cough to expel the object himself.

Choking, conscious, but cannot breathe and is turning blue: This situation requires immediate intervention to expel the object blocking the airway. The following contains a summary of the American Heart Association's guidelines for the modified Heimlich maneuver for infants under age one. Because an infant's organs are fragile, be gentle. Do not use the standard Heimlich maneuver recommended for older children and adults.

STEP 1: Positioning.

Place your son facedown on your forearm in a head-down position with the head and neck stabilized. Rest your forearm firmly against your body for support. For a larger infant, you may instead lay him facedown over your lap, with his head lower than his trunk and firmly supported.

STEP 2: Back blows.

Give four back blows in succession with the heel of the hand between the shoulder blades. Adjust the force of your blows to the infant's size.

STEP 3: Chest thrusts.

If he still cannot breathe, turn him over onto his back, resting on a firm surface and give four rapid chest thrusts over the breastbone, using only two fingers. Adjust the force of your thrusts to your son's size.

STEP 4: Foreign body sweep.

If he is still not breathing, open the airway by using the head-tilt/chin-lift: Place your hand—the one closest to his head—on his forehead. Place one or two fingers—but not the thumb—of your other hand under the bony part of his chin. Gently tilt his head back to a neutral position by applying gentle backward pressure on his forehead and lifting his chin. Do not close his mouth completely.

Look at the airway for a possible foreign body. Do not try to remove the object unless you can see it. If you see it, sweep it out with your finger rather than attempting to grasp it.

STEP 5: Mouth-to-mouth resuscitation.

If he doesn't start breathing on his own, give him mouth-to-mouth resuscitation as follows:

Take a deep breath.

Place your mouth over his nose and mouth, making as tight a seal as possible.

Give two slow, gentle breaths, one to one-and-a-half seconds each, allowing the child's lungs to deflate fully between each breath. With an infant, be careful not to exhale with too much force.

Remove your mouth between breaths and look and listen for air leaving the lungs.

CAR SEAT SAFETY

Once your baby reaches twenty pounds or twenty-six inches and can sit up by himself, you can move him to a forward-facing car seat, but still keep him in the backseat. Front passenger air bags can kill a child when they deploy. If you have any questions about moving from a rear-facing to a forward-facing seat, call the federal auto-safety hotline at 800-424-9393.

STEP 6: Repeat the steps.

Continue to repeat steps one through five until the object is dislodged or medical help arrives.

Physical Growth

Your son will double his birth weight by the time he is four to six months old and will grow about one to one-and-a-half inches each month. Overall, he is beginning to look less like an infant, and more like a person with his own distinctive appearance (a once-bald head may now be showing a bit of hair). By sixteen to twenty weeks, most boys can turn their heads to both sides, and between twenty-four and twenty-eight weeks they'll lift their heads while lying on their backs. Between six and seven months, you'll notice that the muscles in your son's arms and legs are growing quite sturdy (the better to scoot all around your house with!). His body proportions are changing as the lower body becomes bigger and stronger. This will allow him to start rolling from one place to another between eight and ten weeks, and then somewhere between six and nine months to creep on his stomach and drag his legs behind.

FINE MOTOR SKILL DEVELOPMENT

As your son's large muscles are developing to prepare him for action, his fine motor skills are also developing so he can better hold, handle, and manipulate the things in his world.

By six months, most boys can briefly hold onto an object like a small block and will soon learn to bang two blocks together. You'll also see that, although the way he grasps things is a bit clumsy, he is fascinated by this ability. In fact, he'll try to grab anything in his sight—even pictures in a book.

This is also the time when you'll see how much fun learning can be. I remember the look of absolute joy when my six-month-old son discovered that the block he held in his one hand could be dropped into the cup he held in the other. And then came the squeal of delight when he turned the cup over and the block fell out. What a great day for both of us!

By seven months of age, you'll see that he can not only grab and hold an object, but let go of it, too. He can also move the object from one hand to the other. This is quite an accomplishment that he will love to practice over and over again. So keep a few blocks on hand, place them just within his reach, and watch his fine motor skills grow.

Emotional Development

While your son is growing larger in size and physical capabilities, he is also growing emotionally. He is learning about feelings such as accomplishment and security, and he's starting to recognize that he is a separate human being who is very special.

A BABY BOY'S FIRST FEELINGS: FEAR AND FRUSTRATION

Being an infant in an ever-changing world is not always easy. Your son may start to show signs of fear and frustration as he tries to understand his world and often falls short.

Babies develop fears about the most ordinary things. Your son may one day panic when you remove his clothes and he feels discomfort about being naked. Or he may throw a fit when you try to lower him into a warm-water bath. Or he may suddenly become afraid of his stuffed animal. These fears are usually short-lived and nothing to worry about; they are signs that your little boy is becoming more aware of his environment, and the fact that not all of it makes sense to him.

You can help your son get past these fears by accepting them and working to help him deal with them. If, for example, he doesn't like to be naked, keep a light blanket nearby that you can gently put over him, even when you're changing his clothes. If he doesn't want to take a bath, sponge bathe him for awhile. And if he screams every time he sees a certain toy, put the toy away. Don't worry about "babying" him and feeding his fears. He *is* a baby, and right now he needs to know that you respect his feelings and are there to protect him.

This is also a time when your baby boy will get frustrated when he can't do all the things he wants to. If he wants a toy that's just out of reach, he may now scream at his failed attempt to grab it. If he wants the bottle that's sitting on the counter but can't get it himself, he'll let out a howl—not of hunger as he would earlier—but of frustration.

When this happens, it's sometimes best to stand back and watch for a little bit rather than jump to the rescue. If, for example, your son is trying to get a block out of a box but finds that it's stuck, don't help him right away. Give him a chance to work it out, to try harder, to accomplish the task himself. By not running to the rescue too quickly, you teach your son how to handle the frustration that often comes when he is learning something new. He'll eventually learn that if he keeps trying, he'll be successful. This is far better than looking to you solve all his problems.

YOUR SON'S GROWING SENSE OF SELF

Although it's hard to imagine, your son has no idea that you and he are not one and the same person. In fact, babies have no way of knowing that any other people exist separately from themselves at all. A sense of self as a separate body and mind, distinct from others, does not develop until a child is about eighteen months old. Much of life before then is devoted to learning to make this distinction.

This self-awareness begins with a thorough exploration of the body. What a joy to watch a baby this age examine his hands and feet. He stares and studies them for long periods memorizing what they look like and how they work. I imagine he is saying to himself, "What a piece of work I am!"

Your son's increasing ability to control his body movements also contributes to his growing sense of self. As he comes to realize that he can manipulate and interact with his world (by taking off his socks, for example), he gains strong feelings of mastery and accomplishment. Each success contributes to his view of who he is and his value in the universe.

Cognitive Development

Your son is polishing up his thinking skills every time he touches, smells, sees, feels, and tastes his world. Between four and seven months, you'll start to see evidence of all that he's been learning.

WHAT YOUR BABY BOY KNOWS

Watch your son closely as he examines a toy, and you can almost see the wheels in his head turning. You can see him thinking: "If I do this, then that will happen." You can see this cause-and-effect thinking process when he intentionally kicks at an object to make it move. He will slam his open hand on a toy to make it squeak. And he'll even drop his bottle on the floor just for the joy of knowing that you'll retrieve it.

Anticipation is an advanced thinking skill for a little one. You'll see this intellectual feat when you wiggle your finger and move in slowly to tickle his tummy. After playing this game a few times he learns to anticipate the tickle and will squeal with delight before your finger touches his body. You'll also see signs of this skill when he smiles and waves his arms and legs as you begin to prepare his bath. He knows the chance for some good splashing is on its way.

This is also time for some major experimentation. Your son is starting to be interested in how things work and what they do. Watch as he pokes at a toy, bangs another, and shakes a third. He's experimenting to find out which ones roll, which ones make noise, and which ones do nothing at all. Around six to seven months, he'll start to remember how things work, and he'll know in advance that the rattle will make noise and that slapping his hand on the bath water will make a wonderful splash.

You can help your son in his quest to learn all about his world. Because he learns so much by simply watching, give him a change of view every so often. Move him to different places around the room and the house so he can see different perspectives. Take him

EVERYDAY TEACHING TOOLS

Some of the simplest daily activities can serve as great teaching tools. Here are a few to get you started:

- Explain what you're doing as your put the key in the lock to open the door. Point out that the water from the tap can fill up the container.

- Place your baby's toy under the blanket and ask, "Where is it?" He'll eventually learn to look for it and will be delighted by his mastery of this fascinating game.

- When you hear a family member approaching ask, "Who is coming?" When the person arrives, name him or her so your baby learns both to anticipate and to name.

outside, bring him to the park, take him for a walk in his stroller. These experiences are all learning opportunities.

LANGUAGE DEVELOPMENT: LA-LA-LA

Although your son won't be talking for a while yet, he's learning a lot about language. His ability to understand words will be far greater than his speaking vocabulary, so don't assume because your baby isn't talking yet, there's no point in talking to him. During these few months, you'll notice that he will respond to certain familiar words. If you ask him where the dog is, he'll look around for it; if you call his name, he will turn to you; if you ask him where Daddy is, he'll look right at him. There's lots of language development going on before your son says his first word.

Between four and five months your son may make his first attempts to communicate by making the most delightful sound—I call it razzing. He'll blow through his lips, often with saliva bubbles, to make a vibrating sound and then laugh at his accomplishment. If you razz him right back, he's likely to keep the game going.

Around six months, he'll begin to imitate one syllable sounds. This is when you'll swear that your baby called your name: *ma* or *da.* Soon he will put together two syllables, and you'll hear (over and over) his favorite sounds such as *mama, dada, and baba,* as well as repetitive syllables such as *la-la-la.*

This is also the time when your son is learning what words mean. By seven months he will begin to understand specific words that he hears often such as *bottle* or *blanket.* The way you talk to your son will directly affect how well his language skills develop. In fact, the more often you have "conversations" with your son, the more developed the language centers of his brain will become. Try these strategies to improve his language skills:

- **Talk to him.** As you rush through your day, talk out loud and tell your son what you're doing. As you put on his shoes, say something like, "Shoes go on your feet." Even if the words you say mean nothing to your baby, he's learning the sound, pitch, inflection, and rhythm of language.

- **Talk back.** When your baby makes a sound, keep the conversation going. Look at him and mimic the sound back. Let him know you're listening to him and enjoying his attempts at communication.

- **Use precise words to label objects.** Instead of using the general word *toy,* use a specific word such as *ball* or *rattle.*

- **Match your tone of voice to your meaning.** If you use a soft, singsong voice to tell your son, *Don't touch that,* it will be hard for him to understand what you mean. If you are giving a warning, he needs to hear a firm tone that matches the message.

- **Be silly.** Don't worry that your son will pick up bad speech habits if you occasionally use baby talk, singsong words, or even silly, nonsense syllables.

At this age, the most important thing is to enjoy the give and take of communication. Make it fun for your baby to listen and learn.

BABY GAMES

Play is the occupation of children. It is what allows them to grow intellectually as they learn to problem solve (when figuring out where their teddy bear is hiding), to manipulate (when putting a toy held in one hand into the other hand), to learn cause and effect (when pushing a button makes the music play), and so on. So don't wait for your son to be up and running around and making his own fun before you get down on the floor to play with him. Your infant loves a good time and is now ready to show off his developing sense of humor (as you'll learn when he dumps his dish of food on the floor and laughs with glee).

At this age, babies love the anticipation of a surprise. Try the gonna-get-you game by wiggling your finger in the air as you musically say, "I-I-I-I-I'm gonna get you!" And then gently poke your son's tummy and watch him squeal with delight.

Peek-a-boo is another favorite game of anticipation. If you get tired of hiding your face behind your hands, cover a toy and let your child uncover it.

Singing games are always fun for your son because they're repetitive and predictable. "The itsy-bitsy spider" is an old-time favorite with fun hand movements that your son will soon try to imitate.

Body games are always fun. "This little piggy" and "where are baby's eyes, nose," etc are not only good for a hardy laugh, they help your son learn about his body.

Between four and seven months, your son's sense of humor will start to show. A game of peek-a-boo may have attracted his quiet interest in the past, but now will spark giggles with arms and legs waving in joy. And if you have an older child, your son will especially enjoy playing with him or her. One funny face from a sibling can give an infant a great belly laugh. But don't let them play unsupervised. An older sibling can very easily (and unintentionally) harm a baby. It would not be unusual for a three-year-old to wonder if a spoon inserted into the baby's one ear would come out the other side!

ENJOYING A GOOD BOOK

You don't have to wait until your little boy is older to read him a bedtime story. Even infants love a good book. The all-time favorite in my house was a wonderful book called *Pat the Bunny*. My babies loved it because each turn of the page gave them a new texture to feel. They would bang their little hands against the cardboard page and delight in the feel of the soft fur, and then more gently touch the scratchy paper.

While you read to your son, for a short while he will carefully listen to the cadences of your words and phrases with rapt attention. He is learning to speak by listening to your voice as its tone, pitch, and inflection changes.

Reading picture books to your baby also helps him learn about his world. He will enjoy looking at books that have pictures of things he finds in his own world: babies, toys, familiar animals, and vehicles. As you show him these pictures, name them and, when appropriate, make accompanying sounds. If you have a cat in your home, for example, get a picture book about a cat. As you read it to your son, point to the picture and then to your family cat, name the animal—"cat"—and add a meow. There's so much to learn and books are a great way to make that learning fun, even for infants.

Social Development

Infants between four and seven months are very social. You've seen your son bubble with happiness when even a stranger stops to say hello. Each social interaction teaches him that he is someone special and that he can have an effect on the world around him. Having the opportunity to be among people helps your son learn who he is and how he fits into his world.

You might even consider setting up a playdate for your little one. When my son Matt was still an infant, I had a good friend with a son the same age. We often got together for a cup of tea and some adult company. We'd put our boys down on a blanket and turn our attention to our own conversation. It sure didn't look like much was happening between the boys at these little playdates. They lay or sat next to each other and entertained themselves with their own rattles or toes. I didn't realize at the time (but have learned since) that these social get-togethers were just as good for my son as they were for me.

Developmental experts tell us that side-by-side play with other babies gives infants opportunities to get used to being with other children, to watch them, and to imitate their actions. These are important first steps toward learning how to interact with others. Given the opportunity to play with the same child regularly, even infants can become friends.

Get Ready to Run!

Rest time is over. As your baby boy moves into the eight- to eleven-month age group discussed in the next chapter, he's ready to hit the road. He'll be creeping, crawling, walking, and running before you know it—with you right behind him. So get out your track shoes and get ready for some fast-paced adventures.

MY BABY BOY

The best thing about having a boy is: everything! Boys are generally easygoing and let you dress them. (They usually don't have outfit preferences.) They usually don't even need their hair combed, let alone need barrettes, bows, etc.

—Kim Hauser
Mother of Nicholas, age 4½, and Douglas, age 7

Four

Movers and Shakers

Your Boy from eight to eleven months

I will confess right up front that raising my boys from eight to eleven months was a challenge—and that's putting it kindly. From the moment they figured out how to propel their bodies forward, they were both calamities on wheels. There wasn't a cord, curtain, cabinet, closet, drawer, chair, electronic device, or electrical appliance that was safe from their inquisitive explorations. In a moment of desperation, I even wrapped my soft, one-pound exercise weights around Joey's little ankles, hoping to slow him down. Of course this didn't calm my little whirlwind, but I do think it strengthened his legs, making him game for even more risky adventures!

I also remember that this period gave me my first inkling of my boys' unique and wonderful personalities. This was when I first saw Matt's focused intellectual curiosity about everything in his world and his desire for order as he neatly lined up his cooked green beans before eating them. It's also when I realized that Joey had a remarkable sense of humor and that it gave him great joy to make funny noises over and over again to keep me laughing.

You may have to put on your sneakers to keep up with your little boy these days, but also be sure to slow down every once in a while, so you can sit back and admire the unique and grand person he is becoming.

Feeding Basics

Your son's eating habits will dramatically change during these months. His staple diet will move from liquid to solid foods, and he may switch from bottle or breast to a cup. These changes give him lots of experiences with the taste, texture, and enjoyment of food that make for lively mealtimes!

WEANING FROM BOTTLE OR BREAST

There's no rule about when a baby should stop breast- or bottle-feeding. My boys switched to solid foods and a sippy cup around their first birthday, though my daughter clung to her bottle until she was past two. (In fact, when she began carrying around her juice bottle as if it were a favorite blanket, my husband and I decided to "lose" it on a family outing.)

As you begin to introduce solid foods, your son will let you know what he needs. You might find that he does not want to nurse or bottle-feed as often. If this happens, you should cut back one feeding at a time, starting perhaps with a midday meal (because this tends to be the smallest and least convenient feeding).

Most parents hold on to the last feeding before bed for quite a while after the first birthday. Others continue to provide bottle or breast milk "snacks" at the baby's request until he loses interest.

If you are breast-feeding, you may decide at this time to completely wean your son. This should be done slowly so that your breasts have a chance to adjust. If you suddenly stop, they will become engorged with milk and that can be very painful. Cut out one breast-feeding a day at first and then two, and so on. If your son is

WHEN IT'S TIME TO USE A CUP

Here are some guidelines to help you decide if it's time to wean from bottle or breast:

☐ Has your son lost the tongue-thrust reflex that caused him to instinctively push things out of his mouth? Does he easily, without gagging, swallow pureed foods? If so, he may be ready for the switch.

☐ Is your son able to sit up by himself? This is a good indicator that he's ready to sit down for a good meal.

☐ Does your son reach out to grab for food? This could be a sign that he'd like to experiment with non-liquid foods.

not yet one year old, you should switch to formula rather than cow's milk even if you wean him off the breast to a cup.

A TOTALLY SOLID FOOD DIET

Once you have introduced a variety of single foods (as discussed in the last chapter), you can start to mix it up, serving a combination of fruits, cereals, and vegetables (still thoroughly pureed, of course).

When your son can sit on his own and is handling the purees well, you can start offering coarser textures. You can also start offering finger foods. Be sure these are soft and cut into small pieces. He will either swallow them whole or let them dissolve in his mouth. Favorite finger foods include bits of cooked carrots, potatoes, or peas, bits of whole-wheat bread or crackers, and Cheerios or a similar cereal. (At first you'll find that your son smushes, spatters, and throws far more food than he eats. It's all part of the learning process.)

Many children are prone to gagging and even throwing up when they are learning to eat. This may happen if the child has too much food in his mouth or if he encounters a new taste or surprising texture, like a lump hidden in smooth pudding. If this happens to your son, give him only small amounts and continued experiences with foods of different textures. If the gagging reflex continues, be sure to mention it to his doctor at the next checkup.

DRINKING FROM A CUP

This is the time that many babies like to try drinking from a cup with a spouted lid. When you first offer a cup to your son, don't expect a civilized reaction. He will shake it, bang it, and throw it.

So it's best to fill it with just a bit of water at first. Demonstrate how to use it and encourage him to sip from the spout. Once he gets the hang of it, you can then offer breast milk, formula, or water in the cup.

Once your son is eating fruit, you can try fruit juice. But don't overdo it. It's better for tots to learn how to eat fruit (which has more fiber) and drink water (which has no sugar) than to get them bonded to juice (which has a lot of sugar and sometimes causes diarrhea). The sweet taste of fruit juice can seduce some children into becoming habitual high-volume juice drinkers, crowding more nutrition-rich foods out of their diets. A baby of one year, for instance, shouldn't drink more than about four ounces of juice a day. In fact, it's fine for a baby to drink no juice at all, as long as he eats fruit.

For ease of use, try giving your son a two-handled cup, either open on top or with a top containing a spout. Some baby cups have a valve in the spout that prevents spills, allowing the liquid to come out only when the child sucks it. These are neater, but be sure you clean the spout thoroughly. And switch off with other cups so he also gets to sip, rather than only suck.

Bedtime Ritual

My Joey never wanted to go to bed—ever. We'd put him in his crib, tiptoe out, and then brace for the scream that would follow. We'd take him out, bring him to the living room with us, and try again a half hour later. And then repeat the routine again. Finally, we'd let him fall asleep wherever and whenever he wanted. There was no routine or pattern to his bedtime. This was a big mistake that made bedtime miserable for the whole family.

Through my research, interviews, and writings on parenting issues, I've since learned that because babies have no idea when they're supposed to go to sleep, they need us to set the stage and make bedtime predictable and routine. By eight months, your son's biological clock has kicked into gear, so he's certainly ready to respond to a consistent bedtime ritual that is both predictable and soothing and that will help him fall asleep at the same time every night.

A bedtime ritual consists of anything you'd like to do as you routinely put your son to bed for the night. A typical ritual might go something like this: You carry your son to the bedroom, turn

SLEEP-DEPRIVED AND CRANKY

The National Sleep Foundation says that our babies no longer "sleep like a baby." They have found that babies average almost ninety minutes less sleep a day than the fourteen-hour minimum that doctors recommend. It's not that they're going to sleep later or getting up earlier, but rather the quality of their sleep is disturbed throughout the night due to trouble falling asleep, heavy snoring, waking up at night, nightmares, and restless legs syndrome (involving unpleasant sensations in the legs, like itching and tingling). Sleep experts say infants and toddlers need enough sleep to remain alert and open to the world around them, and they attribute the problem to the current hectic patterns of daily life.

on a night-light, sit to sing a lullaby, kiss a few stuffed animals good night, kiss your son, and lay him in his bed. You say good night and leave the room while he is still awake. After doing this repeatedly, your baby will know it's time for bed as soon as you turn on the night-light. Same time, same place, same routine every night. The sameness of the ritual carries comfort, security, and a promise that the separation caused by sleep is predictable and temporary.

Whatever rituals you create, make sure they're ones you can repeat and can pass on to your child's caregivers. If you build a routine that includes a story, a song, and a night-light, your spouse and babysitter will never get your child to sleep if they don't follow the same steps (in the same order). These are signals that tell your son what to do next. Without them, he'll lose his sense of security and control.

Discipline: A Boy's Favorite Word—No!

As your son grows, he'll become more mobile and assertive, though he can't mentally understand consequences or consciously control behavior. He will invariably want to do dangerous or disruptive things, such as pulling on curtains and electrical cords, but he's far too young to be punished. He has no way of understanding why you would slap his hand when he grabs hold of the curtain. He doesn't connect a loud scolding with putting something dangerous in his mouth. And he's certainly too young to obey your "don't touch" warning.

Your best approach in helping your son to behave at this age is to distract him from potentially harmful situations with fun activities, music, or a favorite toy. When you see him cruising toward the electrical outlet, firmly say "no," turn his body around, and grab his attention with a new game or toy. If your son is pestering the family dog, say "no" and then take your son or the dog out of the room. Although your son is too young to completely understand what he did wrong, he will soon learn the word *no*. In fact, "no" is often one of a baby's very first words, soon followed by a shake of the head. At first he won't know what the word means, but because he hears it so often, it's easy to repeat. And it is much easier for babies to shake their head from side to side than it is for them to nod up and down, so he will respond to almost anything you say with what seems like a negative. He's just practicing for the terrible twos when he finally knows what "no" means and likes to use it a lot.

Although your son is too young to understand the consequences of putting his finger into an electrical outlet, he's starting to learn how the things he does affect you. Just to see how you will react, he might experiment with behaviors such as pulling your hair, biting, poking, and high-pitched screaming. If you overreact, you can inadvertently encourage him to repeat the behavior—strong reactions are exciting to babies and experienced as positive reinforcement rather than punishment.

Instead, if your son is screaming just to get attention, ignore him until he stops. When he does, reward him with hugs and kisses. Rewarding good behavior can be a powerful tool for discipline. If your son is biting or poking, stay calm, firmly let him know, "No, that hurts," and restrain him for a few moments. If he persists, put him down for a few moments and then explain your actions in simple words.

You can best lay the foundation for later discipline by showering your son with love and attention. Have no fear—you can't spoil a child this young. Use this special time of infancy to make your child feel loved and important, which will, in turn, teach him about feelings of love for you. By the time your son is a toddler and ready for firmer discipline, he will be more likely to listen because he wants to please you.

Medical Care

Poison, toothcare, antibiotics, ear infections. These months will keep you hopping as you try to give your little boy room to grow, and at the same time keep him safe and healthy.

ROUTINE AT-HOME CARE

Prevention is the key to good health in this time of late infancy. Keeping cabinets locked and teeth polished will head off problems before they begin.

Poison Control: Now that your little boy is finding his way around, you should literally batten down the hatches. The combination of his mobility and his instinct to put everything in his mouth for exploration can be deadly if he consumes a toxic household substance or medication.

To make sure your child isn't one of the 1.2 million children younger than age six who ingest potentially poisonous substances each year, the website www.KidsHealth.org recommends these helpful tips:

☐ Store all medications, vitamins, cleaning supplies, and alcoholic drinks in high (preferably locked) cabinets. Cosmetics and toiletries should also be kept far from children's reach.

☐ Never tell a child that medicine is "candy."

☐ Take special precautions when you have houseguests. Be sure their medications are far from reach, preferably locked in one of their bags or stored in a high cabinet during their visit.

☐ Don't rely on packaging to protect your children. Child-resistant does not mean childproof.

☐ Keep medications and cleaning supplies in their original containers—not in old soda bottles or containers that were once used for food.

☐ While cleaning or using household chemicals, never leave the bottles unattended if a small child is present. Similarly, take special care with alcohol during parties—guests may not be conscious of where they've left their drinks.

☐ Keep rat poison or roach powders off the floors of your home.

☐ Keep hazardous automotive and gardening products in a securely locked area in your garage.

OUT WITH IPECAC

If you have a bottle of ipecac syrup in your medicine closet, throw it out. That's the most recent recommendation from the American Academy of Pediatrics. This syrup has long been recommended to induce vomiting in children who have swallowed poison or accidentally overdosed on medication. But the Academy has cancelled this recommendation because there are some poisoning situations where vomiting can actually be more harmful to the child and because any child who has ingested poison or medication should be rushed to the hospital whether vomiting is induced or not. Instead, it is recommended that parents focus on poison prevention in their homes and keep this number for poison control handy: 800-222-1222.

☐ Learn all the names of the plants in your house and remove any that could be toxic.

☐ Discard used button-cell batteries safely and store any used ones far from children's reach (alkaline substances are poisonous).

(This information was provided by KidsHealth, one of the largest resources online for medically reviewed health information written for parents, kids, and teens. For more articles like this one, visit www.KidsHealth.org or www.TeensHealth.org. © 1995–2004 by The Nemours Foundation.)

ROUTINE CHECKUPS

Your son may look perfectly healthy to you, but he still needs to see his doctor for routine checkups. The American Academy of Pediatrics recommends a well-baby exam at nine months.

Just like the previous health checkups, your son's doctor will give him a complete once over. She will:

☐ Record your son's physical growth: his weight, length, and head circumference will be measured.

☐ Flash a light in his eyes to monitor pupil dilation. She will also move the light from side to side, asking your child to follow the light with his eyes. She is looking to see if they wander, cross, or move in different directions—all signs of strabismus, a common, often correctable, childhood eye problem.

☐ Examine his ears by checking behind the eardrum for fluid; and the middle ear for redness, swelling, or other signs of infection.

☐ Look inside the nose, checking nasal membranes for swelling due to a cold or allergy and the mucus for color and consistency (this may indicate infection).

☐ Ask the baby to open wide to check the mouth, throat, and tonsils for bumps, sores, swelling, or color changes—all signs of infection.

☐ Use a stethoscope to listen to your son's heart for rate and rhythm and lungs for any respiratory problems.

☐ Feel your son's abdomen to rule out abnormal masses or enlarged organs and check for gurgling sounds of the intestinal tract.

☐ Check the genitalia for any signs of tenderness or infection.

This visit also gives you a good opportunity to discuss any health concerns you may have. If you're wondering if your son's physical development, large motor skills, language skills, feeding schedule, or sleeping patterns are on track, ask. Your son's doctors sees many infants every day and cannot know what child development issues are most important to each parent. If at all possible, your partner should also accompany you. This lets both of you get to know the person charged with caring for your son's health. It also offers an extra hand so that at least one of you can listen to the doctor's advice without being distracted.

Tooth Care: By the time your boy is eleven months old, he is likely to have his two bottom and two top teeth as well as his upper and lower side teeth. This is the time for your baby's first visit to the dentist! The American Dental Association and the American Academy of Pediatric Dentists recommend that children see a dentist by age one, when they generally have about six to eight teeth. These dentists say that dental problems in young children may be difficult for parents to spot. Therefore, even though the teeth look fine to you, there may be signs of early trouble that a dentist can detect. Also, a dentist experienced in treating young children can give you extra guidance on how to clean those little teeth and how to prevent future problems.

If you decide to take your child to a dentist at this young age, it's best to find a pediatric dentist who has special training in dealing with children, or a family dentist with a lot of experience with kids. An office that caters to children generally will have interesting toys and books in the waiting room, hygienists who know how to talk to youngsters, and cheerful props and take-home goodies.

This first visit will be for a checkup only. Your son will sit on your lap, and if he hasn't developed a severe case of stranger anxiety just yet, he will probably enjoy looking around at the new environment while the dentist examines his teeth. This should be a pleasant visit without discomfort or fear, which can help him avoid an early case of dentist phobia.

COMMON HEALTH CONCERNS

As you watch your son grow, you will routinely deal with normal health concerns such as sniffles, colds, bumps, and bruises. But when your son has an ear infection, you should visit the baby's doctor for proper treatment, which may or may not include a course of antibiotics.

Ear Infections: Ear infections (medical term: *otitis media*) are the second-most common childhood ailment, following upper respiratory infections. So what causes these common infections?

When a baby lies flat, the Eustachian tube—the tube that connects the back of the throat with the middle ear—is more horizontal. This allows fluid and germs to travel more easily from the back of the throat to the middle ear. This tube is shorter in babies, so the fluid more easily finds its way into the middle ear. That's why if your son has a head cold, it may lead to an ear infection if fluids back up into the ear, giving the germs that cause ear infections a nice warm place to grow. Fluids like formula, breast milk, or juice that he drinks while lying down can do the same thing.

Oddly enough, allergens can also cause ear infections. The allergens in cigarette smoke, for example, trigger secretions that plug the breathing passages and the Eustachian tube, setting up fluid in the middle ear ripe for possible infection. In fact, even allergens from pet dander can trigger secretions that build up in the middle ear and lead to infection.

So, if your son is prone to ear infections: 1) Always feed him upright (at no less than 30 degrees) and keep him upright for at least thirty minutes after a feeding. 2) Keep him away from cigarette smoke. And 3) keep pets out of his bedroom (and, certainly, don't let your son and your pet sleep together in the same room).

Because ear infections are so common in young children, there's a good chance that your little boy will experience this discomfort. You should suspect an ear infection if he shows these symptoms:

- Irritability. Your son may cry and pull on one ear or the side of his face.

- Unwillingness to lie down (this increases the pain).

- Fever ranging from 100 to 104 degrees.

- Balance problems.

If you suspect an ear infection, get your son to the doctor for an accurate diagnosis. In some cases the infection is minor and will heal itself. In other cases there can be dangerous consequences if the condition is left untreated. Let your doctor decide. If there is no imminent danger, it's possible that because of the rampant over-use of antibiotics, the prescribed treatment will be quite different than it was for babies just one generation ago.

The American Academy of Pediatrics and the American Academy of Family Physicians has issued guidelines with a very specific

TO TREAT OR NOT TO TREAT?

Whether you treat an ear infection with antibiotics or not, here are a few tips to help your son feel more comfortable:

- Don't put over-the-counter eardrops or warm water in your son's ear.

- Keep your son in a sitting position as much as possible. Sitting relieves pressure against the eardrum.

- Offer fluids to drink. Swallowing can open the inner ear tube and relieve pressure.

- Offer children's-strength acetaminophen to relieve pain, with the approval of your son's doctor.

definition of what constitutes an ear infection and how to best treat it. Because it has been found that most children with acute ear infections will get better without antibiotic treatment, the guidelines call for watchful waiting. They suggest that physicians give children a prescription for antibiotics only if they don't feel better in two days. Doctors aren't withholding antibiotics in cases where there is clearly an infection and the child is feverish and in pain, or in instances where the baby has a history of ear infections. But if the diagnosis is borderline, your son's doctor may ask you to hold off on the antibiotics.

OVERUSE OF ANTIBIOTICS

The most pressing reason why your son's doctor may hesitate to prescribe an antibiotic even for ear infections is that overuse and inappropriate use has caused this class of medication to lose some of its effectiveness. Newer antibiotic-resistant strains of bacterial infections have emerged. As a result, some commonly prescribed antibiotics are no longer reliable defenders against such common ailments as ear and sinus infections, tonsillitis, pneumonia, and tuberculosis.

Your son is at risk for developing resistance to antibiotics if: 1) he is given many courses of antibiotic treatments to treat frequent illnesses, or 2) if you stop a prescribed antibiotic treatment before completing the full dose. (This allows infectious bacteria that have not been killed to produce antibiotic-resistant offspring, and the child may suffer a relapse that does not respond to the medication.)

To make sure your son takes antibiotics safely, follow these steps:

■ Do not expect your son's doctor to prescribe an antibiotic for the common cold or other viral infections. Antibiotics do not kill viruses.

■ If your son's doctor prescribes an antibiotic, follow the instructions exactly. If the medication is to be given twice a day for ten days, make sure you comply, even if he appears to feel much better.

■ If you miss a dose or two, call the doctor or pharmacist to find out if you should double up, continue anew, or stop completely.

■ Don't keep leftover antibiotics. If used properly, there should be no leftovers, but if there are, you cannot use "just a little" on another occasion without risking the possibility

CHECK THE DOSAGE

The U.S. Pharmacopeia, a not-for-profit organization that promotes standards for medicines, says that each year thousands of children are given the wrong doses of medications. This often happens, they say, because of a simple miscalculation involving the child's weight. The proper doses of most medications are based on a child's age and weight in kilograms. But most of us know our child's weight in pounds. If you divide pounds by 2.2, you will convert the figure into kilograms, and this will help you confirm with your baby's doctor that the weight and dosage match.

of creating a resistant strain of bacteria. Also, antibiotics lose their potency over time.

Physical Growth

If you can hold your little explorer still long enough to take a quiet moment and reflect back on his first year of life, you'll be amazed at what he has achieved in such a short period of time. Most little boys have tripled their birth weight and doubled their height by the time they are one year old. They have developed their neuromuscular abilities from the head down, first leaning to control the head and neck, then the torso. They can now roll over from a lying-down position and push themselves to sitting in an easy, smooth maneuver. Finally they gain control of the lower body as they crawl and prepare to walk. This physical growth and development between eight and eleven months is just fascinating to watch!

CREEPING, CRAWLING, AND WALKING

Babies sure find interesting ways to get around. In the previous chapter we talked about early creeping when some infants wiggle or slither forward on their stomachs using only their arms or elbows, pulling their legs along. Others learn they can more quickly cover a greater distance by rolling. Some scooch forward while sitting, doing what's sometimes called "bottom shuffling." And then there's a whole group who move only backward!

Sometime between eight and eleven months, most babies will

get up on all fours and crawl forward. (Some, like my Joey, will skip crawling and jump right to walking!) Learning to crawl is a real trial-and-error process. At first your son may get himself into the crawling position and then make a hesitant attempt at movement by rocking or swaying forward. When he tries to move, his balance is unstable and he may fall over. Because his control over his arms and shoulders develops faster than his control over his legs, he may find himself crawling backward away from the object he's trying to reach. How frustrating! This can go on for several weeks until his leg coordination further develops.

When your son does get the hang of crawling—watch out! He's like a tornado with knees. Nothing on floor level is safe from his grasp. So, once again, do a childproofing run through by getting down on the floor and taking stock from your child's viewpoint. The greatest danger to crawlers is from uncovered electrical outlets, ungated stairways, and household cleaners, medications, and other toxic substances. You should also secure or eliminate lightweight furniture, hide or secure electrical cords that can be pulled on, and keep valuable and small objects that can be swallowed on high shelves or locked in cabinets. Then stand back. Your baby's curiosity now has motor power!

Although it's important to remove dangerous items, you don't have to clear a path for your baby to practice crawling. In fact, you can enhance his explorations by scattering pillows around the room for him to climb over or around. Put toys in corners for him to discover, and roll balls across the floor for him to chase. This is great fun for him and also good practice for motor coordination.

Most babies will crawl for a while and then practice walking by pulling themselves up on furniture, moving along while holding

BABY NEEDS A NEW PAIR OF SHOES

Now that your son is getting ready to walk by cruising around while holding on to furniture, be sure his footwear helps rather than hinders his progress:

- Wearing slippery socks on smooth surfaces makes it hard for babies to get around.

- Being barefoot gives your son the best traction (as long as he is in a clean, protected area).

- Buy him flexible shoes with smooth soles that won't grip the floor and cause him to trip.

- Don't choose high-top shoes. They were thought to be the best choice years ago, but they limit ankle movement.

- Buy shoes that fit. If you allow too much "room to grow" the awkward feel will make it harder for your son to walk.

- Resist the stylish shoes (like baby cowboy boots) that are not flexible or porous.

on for balance. They'll cruise around the room going from the sofa to the coffee table to the chair. Sometimes they'll let go and stand unsupported until gravity and a shaky sense of balance pulls them down. Soon, they will walk while holding onto you with both hands, and then with only one. Most take their first uncertain steps alone between nine and thirteen months. That's when the fun really begins!

MALE AND LEFTY

As your son learns to grab a crayon and make a few scribbles, you might see that he tends to use the same hand each time. Although only one in every ten kids prefers his or her left hand, the majority of these lefties are male. This may be because of the male sex hormone, testosterone. Researchers think that too much testosterone in a developing fetus can slow left brain development, giving the right half the edge.

Of course your boy won't be absolutely sure about which hand he prefers until he's about six years old, though even at this early age some parents try to influence the outcome. But you really can't. Being a righty or a lefty isn't a choice that your son will make. Child development experts say that our nervous systems are pre-programmed for right- or left-handedness. In fact, they say that pushing your child to use a particular hand—by placing toys in his right hand or correcting him if he opts for his left—can lead to problems later with hand-eye coordination and dexterity. Let your son use whichever hand—or hands—he's most comfortable with.

Emotional Development

Between eight and eleven months, your son will deal with many different emotions. He is now realizing that his world is far bigger than himself and his immediate family—which can be a scary thing. And he's beginning to develop strong bonds to those he loves while becoming fearful of those he doesn't know. Eventually, with your love and patience, he'll grow to feel secure in this great big world.

FAMOUS LEFTIES

If your son is a lefty (which is more likely if there are other lefties in the family), he's in good company. Take a look at this impressive list of southpaws:

Actors
Tom Cruise, Robert DeNiro, Matthew Broderick

Comics
George Burns, Harpo Marx, Jerry Seinfeld, Richard Pryor, Charlie Chaplin, W. C. Fields

Singers
Isaac Hayes, Phil Collins, Kurt Cobain, Paul Simon

Athletes
Lou Gehrig, Sandy Koufax, Jimmy Connors, Babe Ruth

Presidents
Thomas Jefferson, Gerald Ford, Ronald Reagan, George H. W. Bush, Bill Clinton

   And to wrap up the group, we can add, Mark Twain, Picasso, Leonardo da Vinci, and Einstein!

STRANGER ANXIETY

My son instantaneously developed stranger anxiety in church one Sunday morning. There was a kind, elderly woman with gray hair and glasses sitting next to us, and she leaned in close to touch Joey's cheek. He jerked his body away, giving out a howl that stirred the entire congregation. As he calmed down, she tried again and then again, until finally Joey and I had to leave. He wanted nothing to do with this woman and would not give an inch on that decision. I was flabbergasted. (Yes, that's the only word I can think of that describes it.) What had happened to my friendly little boy?

What happened, I later learned, is called stranger anxiety. On the upside of this developmental stage, your son is learning to distinguish himself from others. He is starting to understand that certain people are familiar and safe—his parents, siblings, and baby-sitter are greeted with joyful smiles of recognition. But on the downside, a previously friendly baby who would delight strangers and distant relatives with his winning personality may now decide that unfamiliar faces are scary and scream at the sight of a bearded man or absolutely refuse to be held by Auntie Mae, who wears glasses.

If your son develops stranger anxiety, don't worry that he's becoming antisocial or pathologically shy. It's a phase that will pass as he learns to feel more secure in his world. To get that sense of security, he may want to sit on your lap (and only your lap) when "strangers" are around, or he may hide his face in your shoulder when introduced to new people. If that happens, don't make a fuss. You won't encourage a sense of security by insisting that he let Auntie Mae hold him. In fact, forcing babies to confront their fears at this age makes them more clingy and insecure.

Instead of pushing your son into social situations that frighten him, enjoy his clingy little grip around your neck and gently help him to let go. You can start by getting him out of the house so he sees lots of different people. When you introduce him to someone he doesn't know or feel comfortable with, keep him in your arms and let him get friendly with the person at his own pace (and accept that it may be a very slow pace). Give him lots of praise for his efforts even when he covers his face with his hands to hide.

You can also help by being friendly yourself. When you interact with other people, your little boy is watching you closely. If you smile and appear relaxed when you talk to the checkout clerk at the grocery store or a visiting relative, your son will learn that these people are okay and that he can feel comfortable with them, too. He builds his sense of trust and security with others by observing you. So smile and relax if your son suddenly seems exceptionally shy. It's a sign that he's growing up and learning to be cautious.

SEPARATION ANXIETY

Along with stranger anxiety, comes separation anxiety—yet another pull on your patience. Until your son is about nine months, he has no idea that you still exist when you walk out of the room. No wonder he screams when you try to leave him!

This fear of losing you is called separation anxiety. It causes most children around ten months to become very clingy and fearful of separation. I was so surprised when my outgoing, friendly, and seemingly independent baby boys suddenly became stuck like Velcro to my leg. They followed me everywhere and screamed in panic if they lost sight of me. Although it was nice to feel so loved,

I felt horrible when I would have to rip them off of me. I was working full-time when my firstborn went through this stage. Every morning I would hand his sobbing little body off to the baby-sitter and listen to his screams as I walked back to my car. It was the worst emotional pain I've ever felt.

I felt slightly better when the pediatrician assured me that his dramatic reaction was quite normal and that he would outgrow this stage of intense separation anxiety. He also offered me some tips on how to help my son deal with these feelings. He said it was best not to give in to his fear by spending every moment at home together. "He needs to learn how to be apart from you," the doctor said. "He needs to know that you leave him—and you return."

You can help your son learn this lesson by continuing to play the separation games mentioned in chapter 2. When your son is awake, say bye-bye, leave the room for a brief period of time, and then return with a smile and offer a cuddle. Do this often throughout the day, extending the amount of time you're out of sight each time. If your son immediately cries when you leave the room, try maintaining voice contact while you're out of sight.

When you do leave your child, don't let the separation and reunion become a dramatic scene. Say good-bye with a smile and leave quickly. (No running back to dry those tears and offer yet more reassurances.) When you return, enter the room calmly with a happy face and offer a warm greeting without getting carried away with hugs and tears and a litany of how much you missed him. Tearful, drawn out separations and returns tell your child that separation is a big deal and something to be worried about.

Your son's world is expanding, and he is now able to separate experiences into those that make him feel comfortable and those that frighten him. This is a positive sign of development. But he needs your help to make these emotional adjustments. So try to be patient when he grabs on and won't let go.

Cognitive Development

Your son's intellectual growth marches forward during these months at incredible speed. At this stage, he is the great imitator. He learns to feed himself by watching how others do it. He lets you wash his face with a washcloth and then will want to take the cloth to wash your face in return. He is learning how to use gestures to communicate, and his memory is improving daily (he may now even remember where he left his favorite toy). Every waking moment is a learning adventure.

A DISAPPEARING ACT

Object permanence is an advanced intellectual concept for little babies. Around nine months, they begin to understand that just because an object is hidden doesn't mean it has disappeared. In the past, if you placed a toy under a blanket, your son would turn away assuming the toy was gone. Now, he will pull at the blanket looking for the hidden toy.

This awareness becomes a favorite game. You'll see how delighted your little boy is when he finds a hidden object. He will enjoy placing an object in a box and then shaking the box to make the object "reappear." Games of peek-a-boo and hide-and-seek are also playful ways to teach the reassuring reality of object permanence.

He may not be ready for a neighborhood game of hide-and-seek, but he'll be delighted when you play "Where's the stuffed animal?"

PLAYTIME: BABY'S FIRST PREP SCHOOL

Child's play is your son's first classroom. You can help him develop his intellect by giving him age-appropriate toys that help him use his new ability to sort, organize, and problem solve. These toys do not have to be high-tech electronic computerized devices. Simple sorting and stacking games are plenty challenging for this age group

Between eight and nine months, your boy may become fascinated with an activity board. These games let your son make things happen. If he pushes this button, he'll hear a certain noise. If he moves a lever, an object will pop up. If he puts his finger in any given hole, a particular light will glow. It's like a science lab for your little one.

Between ten and eleven months, he'll be ready for more advanced experiments. A shape sorter, for example, will both fascinate and frustrate him. He will know that the blocks of various shapes go into the box, but at first he will have trouble using brute force when pushing them in the wrong hole. With your help, slowly he will grasp the concept that he will be more successful if he matches the shape of the block to the shape of the hole.

Babies learn by imitating. Slowly and repeatedly show your son how to work these kinds of toys and then give him room to try. Let him feel some frustration before you jump in to help, so he learns the value of persistence. And always give him a turn and then another and another.

TV ALERT

The value of children's television has long been controversial, but here's some news about kids and TV watching that takes the debate in a whole new direction. Researchers at the Children's Hospital and Regional Medical Center in Seattle have found that it's not the content of the TV shows we should be most concerned about, but rather the amount of TV viewing time. They found that very young children who watch television face an increased risk of attention deficit problems by school age. They say that the unrealistically fast-paced visual images typical of most TV programming may overstimulate and permanently "rewire" the developing brain.

These findings were based on astounding study results. Researchers found that for every hour of television watched daily, children ages one to three faced a 10 percent increased risk of having attention problems by age seven. That means that if your son watches three hours of TV a day, his risk of attention deficit problems jumps 30 percent over children who watch no TV.

This is not the first time the negative effects of TV on young children have been noted. Earlier studies found that television can shorten attention spans, affect brain growth, and the development of social, emotional, and cognitive skills. It can also contribute to the epidemic of obesity and aggressiveness. That kind of serious news should be plastered all over every TV sold: WARNING: TV WATCHING CAN BE DANGEROUS TO CHILDREN'S MENTAL HEALTH.

LEARNING LANGUAGE SKILLS

Your son is learning the language much faster than he's letting on. He may only say a few repeated syllables such as *dada* and *mama*, but his ability to understand language is far more advanced. This is called receptive language. It develops long before your son can put his own thoughts into words. With receptive language the two of you can communicate at a fairly advanced level. He'll now do a lot of pointing and gesturing in response to your words. When you say, "Where's Fido?" he'll point to the dog. When he wants to draw your attention to a toy, he'll pick it up and shake it in front of you. This is all part of language development.

If you compare your son's ability to talk with the vocabulary of a little girl of the same age, you may notice that the girl is far more advanced. It's not clear whether girls are born with a genetic makeup that causes them to be more verbal or whether their life experiences encourage this development. But studies do show that they definitely have the early verbal advantage. Boys tend to take in the language and mull it over for longer periods before attempting it themselves.

In these early months, the best indicator of a male's language development is not the number of words he can say, but rather how well he communicates his thoughts, feelings, and needs in other ways. Facial expressions, gestures, and inflection in sounds all communicate. A child who is able to communicate effectively through actions and behaviors at this age is very likely to eventually attain strong language skills, even if he is not saying as many words as the neighbor's child of the same age (especially if that neighbor is a little girl). If your son can point to the toy he wants, he's saying, "Please give me my truck," and that is an early language skill.

Take, for example, the way your eight-month-old lets you know that he wants to keep playing a game of patty-cake. If you stop and he grabs your hands and moves them to indicate he wants to play more, while kicking his legs and making sounds to keep your attention, that's a very clear message he's communicating. He might also reach up to you, as if to say, "Pick me up." Being able to organize this action to tell you what he wants is a very sophisticated form of communication that Claire Lerner, LCSW, a child development specialist with the national nonprofit organization Zero to Three (www.zerotothree.org), feels too many parents fail to recognize for the advanced skill that it is. "Long before a child has words," she says, "watch for his early methods of communication. They are quite amazing."

Rather than count the number of words your son can say when evaluating his language skills, look to see if he is interacting and communicating in a purposeful way—with or without words. That's the real measure of language growth at this time.

Social Development

The way your son responds to family, friends, and strangers is, in part, determined by his temperament. Does he reach out to everyone he meets? Or does he draw back? Is he friendly or sociable? Or does he get upset by new people and places? Knowing your son's temperament will help you better understand why he acts the way he does in social situations.

SCIENCE SAYS

Without siblings to show them how male and female kids act, children have to rely on the mixed messages of their parents. A 1984 study titled "Sex Role Development and the One-Child Family", found that mothers of an only-child son treated the boy a bit like the daughter that she didn't have—encouraging more feminine behavior than mothers who had several children. Fathers, on the other hand, wanted their only-child sons to be even more conventionally masculine than dads with several children. Boys in this predicament apparently decide to go along with their fathers' expectations. Males without siblings report having even more masculine interests and preferences than other boys.

"EASY," "DIFFICULT," AND "SLOW-TO-WARM-UP" BABIES

When at nine months, my son's doctor told me he was a "difficult" child, I thought he was trying to be nice by avoiding words like *impossible*, *unmanageable*, *obstinate*, and *stubborn*. Turns out, "difficult" is a term used to describe a certain temperament. My baby wasn't trying to give me a hard time, and I wasn't to blame for his crabby disposition. If I had understood that at the time, I'm quite sure our early relationship would have been a whole lot better.

There is scientific evidence that infants do possess distinct temperaments that dictate the way they react to their parents, other people, and their environment. In the 1950s, child development researchers Alexander Thomas and Stella Chess began a now-famous thirty-year study out of New York University Medical Center. They followed 133 infants from birth to adulthood and found that children do come equipped with their own unique personalities. Today, most child-development experts agree and find that the most successful and satisfied parents are those who can adjust their parenting strategies to complement their child's temperament.

In this study (and in today's infant population as well) approximately 40 percent of the children were "easy" babies who follow regular schedules, have a positive approach to change, and experience only mild mood swings. Ten percent were "difficult" babies who follow irregular schedules, have intense reactions to change, and experience frequent negative moods. And 15 percent were "slow-to-warm-up" babies, who are cautious, have a mildly negative response to new situations, and need to approach strangers and situations slowly. The remainder showed a combination of temperament traits that did not fit neatly into one of these three categories.

What kind of baby do you have? Take time during this infant period to observe your son and try to understand how he interacts with his world. The following descriptions are from a book I wrote with child psychologist Charles Schaefer called *Raising Baby Right*. They are very general and apply to a baby's most common behaviors:

Difficult Babies: Kick and cry during diaper changes; awake at night three or four times; cry inconsolably during a trip to the supermarket; pull away and scream when a stranger approaches; awake instantly if the phone rings; if hungry, scream frantically before you have a chance to offer food; stop feeding to turn toward a noise; spend most of the day crying.

Easy Babies: Lie quietly during diaper changes; sleep between midnight and 5 A.M.; enjoy a trip to the supermarket and seem interested in the changing environment; smile and reach toward a stranger; sleep through the phone ringing; when hungry, make sucking noises or sucks on his fingers without much complaining; is not distracted from feeding by noise in the room; spends most of the day in a pleasant mood.

Slow-to-Warm-Up Babies: Wiggle and squirm during diaper changes; awake once or twice between midnight and 5 A.M.; will cry when he first enters a store, but then calms down with only occasional whimpers of complaint; will fuss and shy away from a stranger; whimper or cry out if the phone rings while he is sleeping, but will then fall back to sleep; when hungry, will cry on and off until you offer food; will slow the sucking pace if he hears noise while feeding but will then continue.

The advantage in knowing your son's temperament is not so you can change him to fulfill your expectations. Instead, it is in having an opportunity to create a good fit between your temperament and your child's. This becomes especially important when temperament gets mixed up with stereotypical labels that define how a little boy "should" act.

MORE THAN ONE WAY TO ACT LIKE A BOY

What do baby boys act like? Ask a dozen adults this question and you'll find that many will use adjectives such as active, rambunctious, constant motion, loud, mischievous, feisty, and the like. But actually, these are characteristics of temperament that are based on stereotypes that have nothing to do with gender. Although boys do tend to be more active (as we'll see in chapter 5), expecting your son to act "like a boy" is setting you both up for trouble.

Whether your child is "easy," "difficult," or "slow-to-warm-up," the message he gets about whether or not he's accepted and loved comes partly from the way you respond to his unique temperament. Unfortunately, if a child doesn't fit an expected gender stereotype, the response from parents sometimes sends the message "you are not loved unless you act the way I expect you to act."

Let's say, for example, that two parents each bring their ten-month-old boys to the park one day. One little boy is scrambling all around and exploring every in and out of the park. The other is sitting quietly holding his stuffed animal and watching the other children play. If the parent of this second little boy expects boys to be loud and feisty, he or she will think there is something wrong. The parent will push the boy to go play. When the child resists, the parent may show anger or annoyance. The boy will have no idea what he did wrong, but he'll know that something about who he is has upset his parent.

To better understand the way stereotypes can affect the way you raise your baby, child development specialist Claire Lerner suggests these three important steps:

1. Recognize your expectations of a boy. These are not good or bad, right or wrong. They are simply ideas you carry in your mind that cause you to act in certain ways, which can be harmful to your relationship with your child if your expectations don't match his. If you are a very active, athletic person, for example, you may expect your son to be the same, especially because he's "a boy."

2. Understand who your child is. Avoid "boy" labels based on stereotypes and instead tune in to the child's cues: What makes him tick? How does he react to certain situations? You are the one who can best know what his preferences are, what scares him, what makes him happy. Using this information, you can respond to him in ways that effectively meet his needs.

"For children's developing sense of self-esteem and self-confidence, it is critical that they get accepting messages from their parents," says Lerner. "They need to know, even at this young age, that they are okay. That they are not 'wrong' or 'bad' if they prefer to play quiet games rather than rough and tumble ones."

3. Work with both your expectations and his personality. Use what you know about yourself and what you know about your child to find ways that make you both happy without either of you feeling disappointed or shamed. First, encourage your son to explore his world in a way that makes him comfortable. Then, if you'd like your quiet son to be more active and athletic, you can find ways that are not pushy or disrespectful to engage him in those kinds of activities. If he likes to sit and play quietly with a certain toy, you can encourage more active play by making movement part of the game. You might hide the toy and crawl around with your son looking for it. Show him the fun of active exploration by starting where he is and then moving into motion from there. This isn't forcing him to be someone he's not; it's a way to broaden his experiences by showing him ways he can enjoy active as well as quiet play. The key is to do this in small doses without forcing your son against his will to act in ways that meet *your* expectations.

It's easy to get caught up in stereotypes and give our kids labels that make them appear less able than they are. Lerner learned this from personal experience. "My son was a quiet baby who was slow to warm up," she says. "At playgroups he would want to watch, rather than get involved, and my initial reaction was to worry that he wasn't going to have friends and that he wasn't going to be athletic like me. I sometimes felt compelled to force him to join the other children, but I also wanted to respect his personality." Lerner later realized her son just needed more confidence in trying things out on his own. "Instead of being annoyed that he didn't want to go down the slide, I put him on my lap and took a ride down with him so he could experience the joy and the competency of it, and then he was willing to try it himself," she says. "Once I accepted that he wasn't one of the kids who could jump into a new situation full speed ahead, we had a much better relationship."

MY BABY BOY

The best thing about having boys is:

- How they smell after a bedtime bath as they sit on your lap wearing Superman pajamas.

- How they think that someday they will conquer the world single-handedly.

- How they kiss and hug you lots, but only when no one else is around.

—Nancy Finch
Mother of two boys

Enjoy the unique person your son is growing into by putting aside any labels you attach to the word "boy." Encourage lots of experiences that will allow him to develop at his own speed and in areas that he (not only his parents) enjoy.

Full Speed Ahead

Your baby boy is now leaving infancy behind and moving full speed ahead into toddlerhood. But before he goes, he leaves you with a year full of exciting "firsts," magical moments, and memories of messy faces, silly laughs, and sloppy kisses.

Five

A Toddler in the House

Your Boy from Twelve to Eighteen Months...and Beyond

a your son enters toddlerhood, he'll slowly gain the muscle strength and coordination to run, jump, and climb all over his world, and he won't want to slow down and risk wasting a single minute of any day. What a joy to behold; what a challenge to live with!

This is a stage of rapid growth, intellectual leaps, and emotional ups and downs for your little boy that will whiz by in a flash. So take lots of pictures; it's the only way you'll remember all of the wonderful moments you're in for during this precious time.

Active Little Boys

Little boys define the term *constant motion*. By the end of the day I often felt exhausted just from watching my boys run, kick, jump, hop, twirl, tumble, roll, flip, slip, and glide from one side of the room to the other. I signed Joey up for a toddler gym class just so he could have a place to run without banging into things, and it was definitely worth the half-hour drive there and back just to let him expend some energy. Are all little boys really filled with boundless energy?

In the first year of life, boys and girls are equally active. They all kick their arms and legs, roll around, crawl and cruise with equal vigor. But after the first birthday, girls tend to calm down and boys ratchet up the action. Of course each child is unique, and certainly there are some perfectly healthy girls who never sit still and some boys who prefer quiet play to roughhousing. But there are plenty of studies showing that most often it's the boys who have the higher activity level.

Scientists, who are always curious to know why things happen, have conducted some very interesting studies that point to hormones. Although there's no doubt that boys are socialized to be more active by the games their parents and friends play with them, there are some noteworthy studies that say it's highly likely boys are more active due to their hormones.

These findings first come out of animal studies. Juvenile male rodents as well as monkeys show a consistently high level of rough-and-tumble play or play fighting. This consists of boisterous activity with lots of body contact. Juvenile females normally show very little of this behavior. Alice Sterling Honig, Ph.D., professor emerita of child and family studies in the College of Human Services and Health Professions at Syracuse University, believes that all male mammals that are primates have a higher activity level than females. "Go to the zoo," she says, "and you will see the male monkeys climbing around faster and more frequently than females. Their activity level is noticeably higher. The same is true for human males, too."

The cause, say many, may be the level of sex hormones a child is exposed to before birth. Males and females both produce androgens (the male hormone) and estrogen (the female hormone). But as we will see later in this chapter, when talking about gender roles, the androgren levels are higher in males than in females. This increase may be the reason for the higher activity levels in males. Scientists who have studied personality in girls agree. They have found that females born with higher than average androgren levels are more "tomboyish" than other girls and are more active in sports involving rough body contact (and oddly enough, prefer trucks over dolls).

This explains why even the act of coloring was a different experience for my sons than for my daughter. My daughter was perfectly happy to sit down and color a picture. My sons would sit, then jump up, then sit down, then kick their legs back and forth, then move to another chair, then change position to kneel on the chair, then drop the crayons and jump off the chair to pick them up, and then climb back onto the chair, and then break the crayons into pieces, and so on until it was time to move on to another activity.

Discipline: Building a Foundation

My Aunt Ceil tells a funny story about her son Skipper when he was two years old. An elderly woman bent over and asked him, "What's your name, little boy?" and he answered quite confidently, "No-Skipper-don't." My aunt could only assume that because she forcefully said that phrase to him so many times, he thought it was his name! Yes, this is the time when your lovable little boy may just drive you crazy.

It's quite normal for all toddlers to seek out every conceivable danger and do exactly what they're told *not* to do. They have no self-control and no real concept of consequences. Unfortunately all the scolding and disciplining in the world will not make them understand these things until they get a little older.

And the story gets even tougher because you're the parent of a boy. For various reasons little boys get themselves into more trouble than girls. One reason is because, as we've already learned, boys are more active. As Dr. Honig says, "Boys are the ones who knock over lamps, hurl themselves around the room to get to the other side, bang into things, and cry harder." For all these reasons, says Honig, boys, more often than girls, are disciplined, yelled at, and pushed away.

This is the kind of behavior that sure got the attention in my house. Typically, my daughter would be sitting quietly playing with her toys while my son would be running, jumping, banging, and breaking something. Naturally, he was the one I ended up yelling at every hour or so throughout the day.

Dr. Honig also feels that boys are more often scolded because they don't have the expressive language skills that girls have. "This means," she says, "that when the boy is angry, he may not be as ready to find the words to express those feelings. So instead of saying (as a girl will), 'My toy. Give me,' he may grab and hit and get punished."

And on top of all this, we will see later in the section on learning gender roles, boys are the ones who are often starved for attention. Because our culture expects boys to be more independent than girls, we tend to give our little boys just a bit less care and nurturing. We don't jump as fast when they fall down; we don't hug them quite as close when they cry; and we don't sit down and play face-to-face quite as often. And as a result, it has been found that boys seek their parents' attention—often in negative ways that get them into trouble.

AVOID TROUBLE

Because little boys find it so easy to get themselves into mischief, they need our help to stay out of trouble as they walk, run, stumble, and explore the world around them. At this age, the most effective way to keep your son out of trouble is to eliminate temptations. Keep his environment relatively free of no-no's— items such as stereos, jewelry, and cleaning supplies should be kept out of his reach. As my aunt learned, you will not stop a toddler's curiosity by saying, "No, don't," all day long. This is not discipline; it's systematic aggravation.

In situations where your son digs in his heels and is ready for a fight, try distraction before confrontation. Bring out a favorite toy, draw attention to a new activity, put on some dance music. You can also distract him with a hug and a kiss. Toddler upsets are often caused by frustration and are remedied with comfort and reassurance. Very often he'll gladly call a truce and move on without a fight.

SET LIMITS

While working to avoid trouble, you can also teach your son what he can and can't do by setting limits. Limits are rules that give structure to a toddler's world and help him feel secure. Consistent limits teach all children what is expected of them and how they should behave. Although toddlers may not appear to like the idea of rules, without them the world is too overwhelming and uncontrollable. After repeatedly testing you to see if you really mean what you say, your child will like the feeling of being able to count on certain things. The limits you set should always be clear, consistent, and fair.

PRAISE AND PUNISH

The two methods you can use to enforce your rules are praise and punishment. I have found that praise is by far the more powerful enforcer because it gives kids the positive attention they crave.

However, the need for this attention is so strong at this age that your son may learn to misbehave just to get it. That's why he'll act up as soon as you get on the phone. He knows he can't get your attention without making a scene. To him, negative attention is far better than no attention at all. But it's far better to give him positive attention. When you catch your son being good, stop and praise the effort. For example, "It's so nice to see you being good to the dog."

MAKING RULES

Whenever you make a rule, test it against these factors:

- **Limits should be clear.** Toddlers' language skills are still weak. So your rules should not be too long or too verbal. Simply say, "Don't pull my hair. It hurts me."

- **Limits should be consistent.** If you say "no" this morning, and "yes" this afternoon to the same action or request, you can create a problem that will drive you crazy. It's like working a slot machine—your child quickly learns that if he keeps whining and crying, every so often the effort will pay off.

- **Limits should be fair.** If your son continually breaks every rule you make, you may have too many or inappropriate rules. A toddler's memory is just now getting into gear; it's impossible for your son to remember all the dos and don'ts of the world. So limit the number you expect him to remember to perhaps two or three that really matter.

If you do this often, you'll find you won't need to scold him quite so much for mistreating the dog.

Punishment, on the other hand, should be used far less frequently—even though that's the method of teaching good behavior most of us are more familiar with. We can all tell stories about discipline that begin, "When I was growing up . . ." But times have changed, and because we now know that toddlers are unable to make any connection between their behavior and physical punishment, it's usually more effective to think of punishment as an opportunity for teaching a logical and age-appropriate consequence (that does not involve pain). For example, if your son hits another child, hitting him as punishment doesn't make sense and doesn't teach him what he did wrong. Instead, he should be told not to hit and then immediately removed from the play area. If he throws a tantrum out of frustration, he should be helped through the frustrating experience or ignored until he calms down (as explained a little later), not shaken or spanked.

An effective punishment for a two-year-old is a brief time-out to remove him from the center of attention. To get the most benefit from a time-out, choose a location that's away from the action to make your child feel somewhat isolated, but close enough for you to keep an eye on him. If he won't voluntarily go to the time-out chair, lead or carry him to the chair. Expect protests and ignore them. Make your son stay in the time-out chair for just a short time (one minute for each year of age is a good guideline). When the time is up, welcome your child back. Having to sit in a chair may not sound like a very impressive punishment, but remember, more than anything else, your child wants your attention. A time-out takes this away from him.

TAMING A TANTRUM

Setting limits and using praise and punishment wisely is a good start in teaching your son to behave, but unfortunately, it won't be enough to end tantrums. At this age, a child begins to develop a strong sense of self and wants more control over his environment. The conditions are right for power struggles: "I do it myself" or

DIVORCE AND DISCIPLINE

After a divorce, the parent-child relationship often changes. A study reported in *American Psychologist* noted that the custodial parent, usually the mother, becomes stricter and more controlling, while the other parent becomes permissive and understanding, though less accessible. Both parents make fewer demands for children to mature, become less consistent in their discipline, and have more difficulty communicating with their children.

"Give me." When a toddler discovers that he can't do it himself and that he can't have everything he wants, the stage is set for a tantrum. Being tired, hungry, uncomfortable, frustrated, or in need of attention can all also prompt a child to have a tantrum. Growing up can sometimes be just too much for toddlers to bear.

So what should a parent do when a two-foot-tall demon child starts screaming and kicking? Most of us go with one of two common reactions: either give the child what he wants to shut him up, or throw our own angry tantrum right back. In rational moments we know neither of these options is helpful, but when tempers flare, it's hard to know what else to do (especially when the dramatic scene occurs in public—as it most often does).

I'm not saying it's easy, but the experts who have studied how to best control the behavior of a toddler say we should talk to our screaming meanie firmly but calmly. Say, "You will not get what you want by crying and kicking your feet. When you calm down, we'll talk about your problem." Then, they say, we should create some calming-down time by sending him to his room, or to the time-out chair, or by ignoring him. This helps a child feel he has some control over the situation, and it keeps his sense of self and competency intact. I have to admit, when I had the presence of mind and the fortitude to handle a tantrum this way, I got the best results. Even a toddler will soon figure out that there's no point in putting on a show if there's nobody there to watch.

Teaching your son to behave and show self-control is not easy. It is a very slow and not-so-steady process. The key is to be patient and to never tire of repeating yourself. A toddler's memory is not very good. What you explained last week means nothing this week. His impulsive nature makes it very difficult to stop misbehaving even when he does remember the rules. That's why you

FAMILY RULES

When setting rules for your son, keep this list of don'ts in mind:

- Don't make the rules too long or too verbal.

- Don't change the rules; be consistent.

- Don't have too many rules.

- Don't overreact to tantrums with anger.

- Don't give in to tantrums and let your son have what he wants.

- Don't assume that because your son knows something is wrong that he will have the impulse control to resist doing it.

must select a few very important rules and repeat them over and over to help your son eventually learn what's right and what's wrong in the world he lives in.

Toilet Time

We all know that none of our kids will arrive at their high school graduation in diapers. But for some of us, the process of getting them toilet trained can seem so long and difficult that it's almost impossible to imagine that day.

One of the first books I cowrote with Charles Schaefer, Ph.D., was called *Toilet Training Without Tears*. The most helpful piece of information I took from that project was the reassurance that I shouldn't get crazy because my three-year-old son was still in diapers. Sure enough, when he was good and ready, he decided he didn't want diapers anymore and gladly used the toilet.

The decision about when to start toilet training is a very individual one that depends on personal, social, and even day-care factors. But there is no one "right" time. In the 1920s and 1930s, many parents used a very strict and early approach that is far different from what most parents use today. A 1935 publication by the U.S. Children's Bureau suggested that toilet training should begin shortly after birth. "If not," it continued, "it should always be begun by the third month and be completed by the eighth month." Can you imagine even trying that? In the 1940s and 1950s, attitudes became a bit more permissive, and parents were encouraged to wait until the child was eight months old to begin training. Then, when most households had their own washing machines in the 1960s and when diapers became disposable in the 1970s, toilet training moved into the second and third year, when a child is most physically capable of controlling these physical functions.

Here are some general guidelines about timing that may help you better understand your child's capabilities at this time:

One year: A child may attain dryness after a nap. He may show annoyance at being wet at certain times of the day.

Fifteen months: Some children like to sit on the toilet and may pass urine or a bowel movement (BM); at other times they may resist. Their ability to retain urine and BMs has lengthened to a span of two or three hours. However, placing a child on the toilet may cause him to tense and withhold urine, and he may release it as soon as he is removed from the toilet.

One to two years: Children attain nighttime bowel control.

Eighteen months: A child can respond with a nod or shake of the head when asked if he wants to use the potty. This shows that he can now relate the words to the function. He may report accidents by pulling at his pants. Voluntary control may begin.

Twenty-one months: A child reports accidents by pointing at his puddles. He usually tells you after wetting, but sometimes before. He is pleased with his successes, but the number of daily urinations may start to increase and so the accidents may multiply.

Two years: The child has better control and can verbalize his toilet needs fairly consistently. He may go to the bathroom and pull down his own pants. Bowel control may become established as the child attains voluntary control of the muscle that opens and closes to allow elimination.

Two and a half years: The child is able to hold urine in the bladder for as long as five hours. Two-thirds of children will be dry most of the time. Most are partially trained for daytime bladder control, and nighttime wetting may start to come under control.

Three years: The child has few bowel or bladder accidents. He may be dry all night.

Four years: Almost all children have complete daytime/nighttime bowel and bladder control.

Of course, these are just guidelines. As I know from training my own sons, not all kids follow the same time line. Sometimes a child is not physically able to be completely trained "on schedule" because his neuromuscular system is not yet mature enough to perform the way you want it to. That's why it's important to remember that toilet training is not a discipline problem. There is no room for a drill sergeant in the bathroom.

Whenever you decide to help your son use the toilet and whatever method you choose to do that, your attitude toward the process is just as important as your son's. So keep these tips in mind:

- **Be matter-of-fact.** If you can stay unemotional about this developmental step you will give your child the message that the elimination process is a normal and natural one, a fact of daily living—not something supernaturally wonderful nor horrendously awful.

LEARNING TO WIPE

You may have to wipe your son after a bowel movement for quite some time after he has become fully toilet trained. This is because:

A toddler's arms are too short to fully reach the anal area.

Toddlers lack the dexterity needed to wipe thoroughly.

The consequences of an incomplete job are annoying for child and parent alike.

- **Be tolerant.** This will allow you to calmly bear events that are not at all what you had hoped or planned for. When your child sits on the potty for ten minutes with no results, for example, and then soils his diaper thirty seconds after you put it back on him, you'll need lots of tolerance to stay calm and supportive.

- **Be loving.** During the toilet-training period, show your child unfaltering love and affection. Make a point of offering lots of hugs and smiles. Let him know that if an accident happens, your arms will always be a safe place to run to.

Some say girls are easier to toilet train and are ready sooner than boys. That may be, but in my family, one of my boys was far easier and trained earlier than my daughter, while the other son was quite stubborn and delayed. In the end, they all received their high school diplomas without the encumbrance of diapers.

Water Safety

Most little boys love water. They can splash it, slap it, kick it, pour it, and push it all day long, and it keeps coming back for more. Wobbling on their little toddler legs, they boldly enter the pool, lake, river, or tide without a second thought. And that's exactly what makes water play so scary for us as parents. We know the dangers and pray that our child will never be one of the heart-breaking statistics that make drowning one of the leading causes of death among children. Toddlers are especially prone to water accidents because their arms and legs are small in proportion to their body and head, which makes them top-heavy. A toddler who falls down, even in shallow water, will have difficulty returning to a standing position—unless an adult is standing right there to help.

All my adult life I have been a lifeguard and swimming instructor, and so I have a healthy fear of mixing toddlers and water. But I've also learned a few safety tips that have kept my kids safe and may ease your own fears.

BEWARE "SWIMMING" LESSONS

Many experts have mixed feelings about swimming lessons for toddlers. There's no question that all kids should learn how to swim. At this age, however, the primary purpose of the swim lessons should not be to teach swimming skills. Rather it should be to introduce the basics of water comfort and safety. These early lessons can improve coordination skills, provide exercise for young, developing muscles, and set down a foundation for the later development of swimming skills. But they cannot make a toddler a good swimmer.

If you do enroll your son in a swimming class, be sure you understand its limitations. At this age, your son cannot learn to be responsible for himself in the water. So don't let a false sense of security lull you into thinking you can now read a magazine while your son plays in the water.

PLAY IT SAFE

While close supervision can prevent most water accidents, even the most attentive parents sometimes find themselves faced with a water emergency. In my experience, you can reduce the likelihood of having a bad experience if you follow these simple rules:

- Don't expect flotation devices to keep your child's head above water. The majority of these devices, such as tubes and water wings, are toys and are dangerous if used as any-

SANITARY SWIMMING

Ever notice that the water in kiddie pools is suspiciously warm? There's no doubt that all those little boys and girls are peeing in the pool. But urine generally doesn't spread illness. It's the bowel movements you have to worry about. Even in chlorinated pools, children in diapers can spread infection. So think twice before you allow your child in a kiddie pool full of diaper-wearing tots.

thing else. A child can easily float into water over his head and then fall under using these devices. Even in shallow water, kids who fall down can actually be prevented from getting their heads above the water line because they're wearing these blow-up toys.

- Be especially cautious when your son is surrounded by older children. A toddler who is standing at the water's edge with older kids looks safe enough, but too often the little one is unintentionally knocked into the water. In the excitement of a game, no one may notice.

- Don't count on the lifeguard to watch your son. No matter how many guards are on duty, no one is assigned to watch your child. A lifeguard's job is to look out for major problems in a large group and keep the area safe to prevent water accidents. They are not baby-sitters.

WATER GAMES

The surest way to enjoy your time by the water is to get right in with your child. Your toddler loves to mimic you, so laugh a lot so he can see that you're having fun, and praise his every effort. Here are a few simple water games that I've used in my classes to give very young children a foundation for learning basic swimming skills:

Ping-Pong chase: Have your child blow at a floating Ping-Pong ball and chase it across the water. This game brings the child's face close to the water's surface and gets him ready for bubble blowing.

Ball throw: Throw a ball up into the air and let it gently splash down in front of your son. The water will splash in his face, and when you laugh, he'll learn that water is fun.

Washboard: Hold your son up in the air with your hands under his armpits. Then lower his body down into the water just a little bit. Now lift him back up and down again. Each time you lower him, submerge a little more of his body until his chin touches the water. (Never throw a baby up into the air. Because a baby's head is proportionally heavier and larger, there is danger of injury to the cervical area of the spine.)

Ring-around-a-rosy: This game is just as much fun in the water as it is on land. On the phrase, "We all fall down," your toddler might, at first, lower just his shoulders into the water. The next time, maybe his chin, and so on, until he plunges all the way under.

Use your imagination to make up lots of water games that you and your son can play together—*together* being the operative word. You'll have plenty of time during other summers for beach reading and sunbathing. But for now, enjoy this special time when your child needs your undivided attention in and around the water.

Medical Care

One of the most important jobs of parenthood is keeping your child safe and healthy. During these toddler years, this job alone will keep you hopping. Gone are the little baby food jars and the bottle—bring on table food (and unfortunately, the junk food, too!). Your son's doctor will continue to monitor his growth and health at routine checkups where she will be particularly alert to any signs of food allergies or developmental delays. Here are the details.

ROUTINE AT-HOME CARE

Introducing your son to table food is a fun and challenging experiment. It often takes a lot of time and patience to find foods that are good for him and that he'll actually eat. Good luck!

Eating Like a Big Boy: Your son is now ready to sit with the family and enjoy table food for three meals a day. Although your one-year-old may still be getting half or more of his daily calories from breast milk or formula, regular table food will help round out his diet.

Formula-fed and some breast-fed babies can now switch to cow's milk (unless there is some reason to suspect an allergy). Because babies need fat in their diets for development, most doctors recommend that they drink whole milk until they are two. Then, if their growth is stable and steady, they can switch to a low-fat or nonfat milk.

Although your son is now at the family table, don't expect him to eat like an adult. He will usually eat only a small portion (and play with the rest). He may choose one favorite food and refuse to eat anything else (and that favorite food may change every few days). Most toddlers are quite finicky and often find new foods scary.

If you fight with your son over his food choices, you'll soon find it's a battle you won't win. It's best to offer a variety of nutritious foods and let him take the lead. If he refuses to eat anything but oatmeal cookies for a week, it won't hurt him (as my healthy son can attest to). If he'd rather snack on good foods throughout the day instead of sitting for three meals, that's okay, too, for now. Give him time to get used to good foods and a regular feeding schedule.

Excess weight: As your son begins to toddle around, you may notice that the "baby fat" on his cute little pudgy legs is no longer looking so cute. Once kids are up and about, it gets easier to see that some one- and two-year-olds are already overweight, joining

CHOKING HAZARDS

Before the age of 5, *do not* serve your son the following foods whole:

- hotdogs, especially when cut into circular pieces
- popcorn
- hard candies
- gum or jelly beans
- whole grapes
- raw vegetables, such as carrots, that are cut into circles
- spoonfuls of peanut butter or raw nuts

the whopping 30 percent of all kids who weigh far too much for their age and size—that's triple the percentage of overweight kids from just twenty years ago.

And many children go beyond being overweight. Even toddlers in the United States are obese (defined as being in the 85th percentile for weight), and are showing early signs of diabetes (such as insulin resistance), heart disease (with their elevated blood fats, called triglycerides and low levels of good (or HDL) cholesterol), and other diseases associated with being fat.

As your son begins to eat table foods, now is the time to prevent health problems down the line due to excess weight. But before you put your son on a diet, talk to his doctor. Little growing bodies need an ample supply of protein, vitamins, and minerals that can be limited on low-fat or any of the popular adult diets. You can safely help your son meet his body's needs while staying in shape by following these guidelines:

- ☐ **Set a good example.** Your toddler loves to imitate you, so use that to your advantage. If you choose a piece of fruit for dessert rather than a bowl of ice cream, suddenly fruit will be your son's new favorite dessert, too.

- ☐ **Control portion sizes.** Rather than dish out food family-style from bowls placed on the table, portion out servings on each family member's plate. Offer seconds only of lower-calorie, high-nutrient foods.

- ☐ **Offer lots of water.** Instead of high-sugar juice or soda, offer water or no-calorie, fruit-flavored seltzer.

☐ **Limit fats and sweets.** Don't declare all fats and sweets off-limits. You'll only make them more enticing. Instead, find ways to substitute—an ice pop for ice cream, gelatin for pudding, macaroni with low-fat cheese for lasagna, a poached egg for scrambled eggs, turkey for ham.

☐ **Limit TV time.** Sitting in front of the TV (and munching on junk foods) is a major reason for the rise in childhood obesity. Set a limit and get your son up and moving.

☐ **Increase physical activity.** Toddlers rarely sit still, but often it's more fidgeting than moving. Make sure your child gets time every day for real physical activities, like running and jumping, for at least thirty minutes.

These suggestions are good for the whole family. So do not tease or embarrass your son by saying, "You're getting fat so you can't have ice cream." He can learn positive, valuable lessons about health that will last a lifetime, if they are taught with love and support.

ROUTINE MEDICAL CHECKUPS

Your son's doctor will want to continue to monitor his health and physical development with regular checkups. Most doctors will schedule these visits at twelve, fifteen, eighteen and twenty-four months.

The checkup will follow the same routine as earlier visits with a careful recording of weight, height, and head circumference. The doctor will again check the eyes, ears, nose, and throat. And she will listen to the heart and lungs. She will feel the abdomen for enlarged organs and examine the genitalia for normal and healthy development. And inoculations will be given as needed.

Now the doctor will also tap your son's knees, shins, and elbows with a rubber hammer to check his jerking reflex. This tells her if the brain is sending messages properly down his spinal cord to the rest of his body.

The doctor will probably also ask your son to walk a straight line and jump up and down. This lets her evaluate the child's sense of balance and coordination.

She may also ask your son to touch his toes while she examines the alignment of the spinal cord. A curved spinal cord can indicate scoliosis.

When the exam is finished, be prepared with your list of questions. There's so much going on during these toddler years that it's hard to keep track of all your concerns, so write them down and then ask questions about them. This is a time when lots of parents wonder if their child is "on track." Is his language progressing as it should? Does he have good large and fine motor coordination? Is he really as smart as I think he is?

COMMON HEALTH CONCERNS

The number of toddlers with food allergies is ever increasing—a good cause for concern as your son begins to eat "big people" food. And because your child is a boy, you should keep a particularly close eye on his mental and physical development.

Food Allergies: We all know kids with food allergies—they seem to be very common in today's generation of children. According to the Food and Drug Administration, up to 6 percent of children in the United States under age three have food allergies.

An allergy develops when the body's immune system mistakenly views food as harmful and produces antibodies to help fight off the invader. These antibodies release chemicals that trigger an allergic reaction minutes to hours after the food has been eaten.

Doctors can't predict which children will have these allergies and which ones won't, but there are various factors that place your son at risk. If you or your partner have a history of food allergies or suffer from other allergies or eczema, your child is more likely to develop allergic reactions to food (although some allergic children have no family history at all). Also, if your son has asthma, he is more likely to develop food allergies. And finally, children who

COMMON CULPRITS

A child can develop an allergy to almost any food, but the foods that most commonly trigger allergic reactions include:

- eggs
- fish
- milk
- peanuts
- shellfish

- soy
- tree nuts
- citrus fruits and juices
- wheat
- corn

are exposed at a very early age to foods that commonly trigger allergies increase the risk.

The symptoms of a food allergy range from a mild rash to life-threatening anaphylactic shock. If you suspect your son has had a bad reaction to food, tell his doctor. It's important to identify and avoid the offending food as soon as possible. Repeated exposures to an allergy trigger can make the allergic response more severe and more likely to be a lifelong one.

Of course, severe allergic reactions need immediate medical attention. You should call your doctor or 911 if you see these signs:

- red, itchy rash, or hives

- stomach cramps, vomiting, or diarrhea

- wheezing or shortness of breath

- feeling of light-headedness

- feeling of warmth, flushing, or tingling in the mouth

- severe sneezing

You can reduce the risk of food allergies by withholding common allergy triggers until your child's immune system has had time to mature enough to withstand the offending substance. Gradually introduce the common allergens listed earlier and watch for any signs of an allergic reaction. Wait until your son is two years old to introduce eggs, and hold off on introducing shellfish and peanuts until age three. Even if you've already given your son these products without a problem, it's best to avoid them in the future. Just because your child may have eaten peanut butter without an allergic reaction doesn't mean it still can't happen. Often the body reacts the second or third time a food is eaten.

If your son does develop a food allergy, your doctor can help. Although there is no cure for food allergies, there are medications to treat both minor and severe symptoms. The doctor will also advise you to steer clear of the offending food for a few years. Many children outgrow their allergies, provided that they are not regularly subjected to the food during early childhood.

DEVELOPMENTAL DISORDERS AND DELAYS

When Boys Are the Weaker Sex: We tend to think of males as the stronger sex, but in the early years, just the opposite is true. Males are more likely than females to suffer from birth defects and various developmental problems. In many cases this is because males are at greater risk of being affected by genetic damage. A male has only one X chromosome, and if that chromosome contains damaged genetic material, he does not have another that can compensate, as females do. Even if the defective gene is not immediately life-threatening to the male embryo, other functions may still be affected.

There are approximately five hundred X-linked hereditary diseases affecting boys almost exclusively (girls are usually only carriers). The more common ones include color blindness, hemophilia (a clotting disorder causing excessive bleeding and bruising), muscular dystrophy, and X-linked mental retardation. These are found more often in males because there is no second healthy X chromosome to cover for the defective one. For example, if a male baby has an X chromosome from his mother that contains defective genetic material, he may have hemophilia. A female baby with the same defective X chromosome from the mother would probably have a healthy X chromosome from the father to compensate.

In addition to suffering more from sex-linked genetic problems, in the first year of life males are more vulnerable to infections, learning disabilities, and developmental delays. (In fact, three times as many boys have learning disabilities than girls.) This is why your son's doctor will carefully monitor his development.

We all know we shouldn't compare our child to other children because each one is unique and will develop at his or her own rate. But . . . we all do. And we can't help but worry when our neighbor's child is walking at eleven months and our thirteen-month-old is still scooting around on his rear end. My own sons taught me to be cautious when comparing one child to another. Joey was up and walking with confidence at ten months; Matt took his time and walked at fourteen months. These kinds of perfectly normal delays occur in many areas of development including motor, language, social, and thinking skills and are often no cause for concern.

But if you notice that your son is lagging behind other toddlers in his abilities, talk to his doctor. You'll either get reassurance that everything is just fine, or you'll get early intervention that can keep a small problem from becoming a much larger one. Early intervention is designed to identify and treat a delay in a child as early as possible. The sooner a developmentally delayed child gets proper help, the better his progress will be.

Today, the medical community is finding more and better ways to help babies and toddlers benefit from early help. These services range from early speech therapy or eyeglass prescriptions to a complete program that can involve physical and occupational therapy.

Physical Growth

While your son's developmental growth is moving ahead at an astonishing speed, his physical growth slows down after the first birthday. In the first year, he probably tripled his birth weight, but will now gain only between three and five pounds during his second year. Instead of rapid advances in weight and height, you'll now see changes in his appearance. His rounded belly and soft arms and legs will begin to trim down and become more muscular as he grows from a baby to a boy.

GET UP AND GO

Most kids are competent walkers between thirteen and nineteen months. They then quickly turn into speedsters who run, rather than walk, to every destination (or just for the pure joy of running). Looking ahead by age two your son's large motor skills will continue to amaze. He will be able to climb stairs holding on to a banister with one hand while putting both feet on each step before moving on to the next. He will become extremely good at climbing and will be able to kick and throw a ball (although still rather clumsily).

His fine motor skills are also developing, giving him greater control over his world. As you'll quickly learn, the ability to use

TOYS FOR ACTIVE BOYS

The best toys for this age group are ones that exercise large muscles (and expend all that energy!). For outdoor play, give him toy ladders to climb, wagons to pull, and toy lawn mowers to push. Toys that he can ride on will also be a favorite and will help develop strength and large muscle coordination.

his thumb and fingers in a coordinated way will soon let him twist knobs and dials, push levers, and open drawers.

His improved fine motor skills dictate the kind of toys he will like to play with. He can better grasp a crayon and will make actual drawings with recognizable shapes (especially circles). By age two, he will carefully stack blocks, and with supervision, can fold a sheet of paper, string large beads, manipulate snap toys, play with clay, and pound pegs. You can use these kinds of activities to get your son to sit still for a few minutes of quiet play before he jumps up to again practice those large motor skills of running and climbing.

Emotional Development

Are boys really tough? Not when it comes to their emotions. They feel joy and sadness just as deeply as girls (some say, even more so). Your job right now is to give them the freedom to feel insecure and sad without feeling guilty for being a "sissy."

FOR SECURITY SAKE

My son Matt had a security blanket that I'm quite sure delayed his ability to walk. His early attempts to toddle were constantly sabotaged because he kept tripping over the blanket. One day I brought Matt to the baby-sitter and accidentally left the blanket at home. His frantic screams pushed me to drive all the way back home, retrieve the blanket, and arrive late for work. That night, while he was sleeping, I gently took the blanket, cut it in half, sewed up the cut edges and threw one half in the washing machine. That way I had a small spare piece of the blanket to keep in the car. Matt didn't complain at all about the shorter, cleaner blanket. Over time, I eventually cut the blanket into shorter and shorter sizes. His walking skills improved, and his sense of security stayed intact.

If your son is dragging around a security blanket or a favorite stuffed animal, he has found a way to bolster his sense of emotional security, especially when you're not around. This, child experts say, is not a weakness; it is an early coping skill. If your child is attached to a "banky" or special "friend," don't discourage it or "lose" it when he's not looking (a real temptation when it becomes worn and tattered). He will give it up himself when it no longer serves an emotional need—although he may still want it nearby at bedtime for years to come.

BIG BOYS *DO* CRY

After all the research I've done investigating the differences between boys and girls, I'm going to have to side with those who believe that the sexes are indeed quite different. However, on the issue of crying, there is no debate that little boys do, and should, cry when they are hurt or unhappy.

During toddler years, whether society likes it or not, little boys do cry. In fact, they cry more often and with more force than girls. Most often their tears are shed out of anger or frustration. They cry vigorously to protest being separated from their parents. They cry when things don't work as they should or when their routines are disrupted. Combined with kicking a door or hitting the wall, these tears help boys voice their complaints.

Girls, on the other hand, are better at complaining with words (often very loudly), but cry more often than boys when they are hurt or need help. Some feel this is because girls are better able to use words to express their feelings, but are more dependent on adults for help and direction.

Whatever the reason, your son is bound to cry. It's part of being a person with feelings. When that happens, don't make light of those feelings by telling him, "Oh, that doesn't hurt," or "Be a big boy and don't cry." Instead, try to understand how he feels. The next time your son cries, try something like, "That must upset you very much. Let's see if a hug will make you feel better."

Cognitive Development

Although boys are just as intelligent as girls, their cognitive development progresses at a different pace. Your son has a better grasp of spatial relationships than girls of the same age, but he may not be quite as verbal. However, his budding imagination will help him balance the two as he guides his toy cars through make-believe traffic and practices putting put his abstract thoughts into words.

BOYS AND THEIR LEGOS

Legos and Erector sets might seem like gender-neutral toys, but experts say they're not. Boys show far more interest than girls in these kind of building toys for a very specific reason—boys have advanced development in certain areas of the right hemisphere of the brain, giving them stronger spatial abilities. This means they have a better grasp of shapes and forms, making them more adept at measuring, mechanical design, geography, and map reading.

And get this: It seems that this ability is inborn. Even male rats and monkeys are better at finding their way around than the females. Studies have found that male rats tend to use geometric cues to find their way in a maze, while the females less successfully use landmark cues. Other researchers working with monkeys found similar results with spatial tasks that require them to solve problems by rotating cubes. These studies and many others like them indicate that male superiority in spatial skills is found among all mammals. Perhaps long ago it was the result of necessity. In their long evolutionary history, males generally traveled long distances to find food or mates, or were responsible for guiding a family group. Survival depended on their ability to make their way without confusion.

The next time you see your son happily building a tower out of blocks, keep in mind that this ability comes from thousands of years of evolutionary need. Because he's good at it, he'll prefer it over other games that are more difficult for him.

THE STRONG, SILENT TYPE

The games your son will steer away from will often be the ones that require left-brain action. The left hemisphere of the brain is more active in females, making girls far better at listening, communicating, and all language-based learning. This is probably why men are described as "strong, silent" types.

But this doesn't mean your son isn't interested in communicating with you. He just needs a little push. Most babies say their first true word at one. (Although *mamama* sounded like an attempt at your name, it was just a fun repetition of syllables.) Now you'll hear real words that refer to food (bottle, cookie), people (Mama, Dada, and the child's own name), and toys (ball, doll). At first, your son will use very basic word choices: He will say "dog" rather than "poodle." He will say "flower" rather than "tulip." And he will overgeneralize: All men may be "Daddy," and all round toys are "ball."

Looking ahead, your son will have a vocabulary of between fifty and five hundred words when he is between eighteen and twenty-four months (notice the spread—kids are all unique), and at some point he will string his first sentence together. The thoughts in these sentences may not be profound (in fact, the sentence will probably be just two words long), but the accomplishment is a major advance in learning the language. So listen carefully. One hectic evening, I announced to no one in particular that dinner was ready, and from the other room I caught my two-year-old saying, clear as can be, "Daddy, come eat." To me it sounded like a complete recitation of the Gettysburg Address!

After your son uses two words together to make a sentence, his language growth may explode. The sentences will become longer, and he will soon add pronouns, plurals and the past tenses of verbs. "See truck," becomes "I see truck." "I walk" becomes "I walked." These seemingly minor changes are giant steps forward.

This is also the time when your son's speech will mirror his growing independence. Most children quickly learn to say "No," "Mine," and "Me do it," and they practice these words all day long. Try not to interpret the "no" response as a sign of total negativity. Sometimes, it's just a fun word to say. (Interestingly, toddlers use the word *no* many months before they can use the word *yes*. But you probably already know that!)

Although language skills take giant steps forward between twelve and twenty-four months, there is still a lot to learn. You'll hear your son use pronouns and verb tenses quite creatively when he says, "Us go now," and "Truck comed." But these "mistakes" are all part of learning the language and are no cause to worry.

You can help your child master the English language by trying some of these tips offered by child psychologist Charles Schaefer:

- Fill in the blanks. If your child says "Truck coming," you might reply, "Yes, a big truck is coming."

- Add more information. "That's a big delivery truck."

- Use prompting to encourage vocabulary growth. Say, "Here comes a big " and let your child fill in the blank.

- Have conversations. When you talk to your child, leave a pause, giving your child a chance to respond.

- Ask our child questions (such as "What?" "Where?" "When?") that require more than a yes/no response.

- Label things in the environment. When you visit a park, talk about what you see: "Look at the see-saw. I see a white swan."

- Play language games. These include playing telephone, naming pictures in a magazine, and enjoying nursery rhymes and songs.

- Simplify your speech pattern. While your child is learning the basics, use simple sentences and speak a bit more slowly than you normally do.

- Read! Children learn about language by hearing it.

- Avoid correcting grammar mistakes. Simply repeat the thought correctly. If your child says, "Truck comed," you can say, "Yes, the truck came."

AT HIS OWN PACE

Try to resist the temptation to compare your son's verbal skills with other children (especially to little girls, who are bound to out-talk him). All children learn language at different rates and in different ways. Some say their first word at seven months; others wait until well into their second or third year. There is no definite time line your child must follow. If your son is not saying any single words at age eighteen months or has a vocabulary of less than ten words at twenty-four months, you should mention this to his doctor at his next checkup. But all speech development guidelines give only a general idea of what to expect.

- Don't let your son use pointing as his only method of communication. When he points to the cookie jar, for example, say, "Do you want a cookie?" or "Can you say 'cookie'?"

- Language development often moves two steps forward and one step back. So don't be upset if your son "forgets" the words he knew yesterday.

LEARNING TO PRETEND

At breakfast he is a superhero. By lunch, an astronaut. And after dinner, he's riding his horse off into the sunset. Don't you just love the imagination of little boys?

At this age, children are very imaginative—but they are not born that way. The ability to pretend is a mental skill that develops slowly at the same time a child begins to speak (typically between twelve and eighteen months).

The first signs of your son's imagination will be fleeting: lifting a toy cup to his mouth or a toy telephone to his ear. But soon, he'll be feeding his teddy bear and sitting inside a cardboard "house" with glee. By his second birthday, he'll be mimicking your every move while pretending to clean the house, drive a car, or unsteadily clomp around in high heels.

These imaginary moments are more than just pretend fun. The growth of a child's imagination moves him though many important development processes. For starters, pretend play lets your son explore his emotions. He can express anger by hitting a doll rather than a playmate. He can cope with fear by making his stuffed animal cry, rather than himself. He may practice love and tenderness by hugging and rocking a doll. And you may catch him working through his emerging understanding of right and wrong by scolding his stuffed rabbit.

Pretend can also improve his language skills—especially important for boys. Language uses words to represent real-life objects. So when your child makes a shoebox represent a car, he is developing the ability to think in terms of signs and symbols. Knowing how symbols work is a key factor in learning letters and numbers later on.

The list of benefits from pretend play is quite long. Pretending can enhance a child's self-awareness, self-confidence, and self-control It has also been found to have a positive influence on a child's memory, language skills, and role-taking abilities. That's a lot of benefit from child's play.

Here are a few ideas that will help you encourage this wonderful gift of childhood:

- **Don't discourage your son from using "girl" toys.** In the world of make-believe, dolls and dress up are for everyone. Boys shouldn't be deprived of the benefits of learning how to love or feel grown up "like Mommy."

- **Give your son toys that mimic the real world.** These include toy kitchen utensils, tolls, garden equipment, and dolls.

- **Resist the temptation to substitute real for imaginary.** If your son is pushing a box around pretending it is a car, don't replace it with a toy car. If he uses a banana for a phone, go along with him without pointing out, "That's not really a telephone."

- **Hold back, even when you can do it better.** You may know how to play house better than your son, but let him work it out for himself.

- **Don't correct your child's "mistakes."** If he colors a picture of an elephant pink, purple, and orange, there's no need to point out that these animals are really gray.

- **Let him take the lead.** If your son wants to play school, let him decide who will be the teacher. If he wants to play dress-up, let him choose his outfit.

IN THE TOY BOX

Those expensive toys that claim to make your child smarter are a waste of good money. That's the opinion of the child development experts I've spoken to. This is an age when children learn by imitating, by experimenting, and by doing.

Fill up the toy box with classic learning tools. These include blocks, dump trucks, stuffed animals, and objects that imitate "real life" such as toy hammers, play food, and miniature lawn mowers and doll carriages. Simple problem-solving toys such as shape sorters and nesting cups are also favorites of kids this age as learn how things fit together.

After eighteen months, creative toys will be a hit. Stock up on Play-Doh, crayons, and finger paints. And throw in toys that let your son exercise his imagination: dress-up clothes, action and animal figures, dolls, and stuffed animals.

- **Get him out into the real world.** A dump truck or plastic farm animal can't spark imaginative play if your child has never seen a construction site or a farm.

Social Development

Most toddlers are very social little people. They love to be out and about and are very happy to be with playmates their own age. However, they are quite short on social graces. During this period, your son's behavior is naturally self-centered. He views the world according to his own wants and needs. So don't expect him to share or consider other people's feelings before he acts. Because he still hasn't formed a clear boundary between himself and the outside world, he sees all property as an extension of himself. To him, the word sharing means, "It's mine." This is why true friendships are very rare at this age. Still, this is the time when the foundation for friendships, peer relationships, and cooperative play is established—with your help.

MAKING FRIENDS

Whether your son is the silent, "play by myself" type or the "everything here is mine so stay out of my way" type, he needs lots of opportunities to interact with other toddlers to learn how the give and take of friendship works. If your child is not already in a nursery school setting where he has already learned to fend for himself, playdates are a good way to introduce and practice social skills.

Putting a bunch of toddlers together in one room is a setup for disaster if you don't think ahead. More than once, I opened my door to toddling neighborhood kids and quickly found myself in the midst of crying kids and broken toys. Soon, I learned to get organized.

In the beginning, it's a good idea to limit the number of playmates. One or two friends is plenty. And it's also a good idea to invite the child's parent to stay, too, if he or she has the time. Many children this age still want their parents nearby, and their presence raises the comfort level and reduces emotional meltdowns.

Even with advance planning, kids will fight over toys. When this happens, wait a few moments before stepping in to resolve the dispute. The experience of pushing and pulling until someone wins the toy is often the first stage of leaning how to negotiate. If it

PLANNING FOR PLAYTIME

Playtime will go more smoothly (although never completely without upset) if you think ahead about the toys you'll offer:

- Beforehand, allow your child to put away treasured toys that cannot be shared. Children have a right to a sense of ownership.

- Select toys for sharing that you have duplicates of: trucks, coloring books, blocks, stuffed animals, and the like.

- Plan games and activities that can be played side by side, and rather than put all the blocks (or whatever) into one large pile for sharing, offer each child his own set. This will cut down on those conflicts of ownership.

looks like the battle is going to escalate out of hand or someone is going to get hurt, it's time to distract the combatants. Bring out a new toy or change the activity. If your child can't be distracted, don't punish him for not playing nicely. Instead, remove him from the fun for a few minutes so he can calm down, and then go back and let him try again.

If you step in before the fight gets out of hand, you can sometimes introduce the idea of sharing. It won't work if you say, "You must share!" or "You shouldn't grab toys away from another child." Given his level of cognitive development, your son won't understand why he shouldn't misbehave—it'll go in one ear and out the other. Instead, first acknowledge his feelings, then make a suggestion: "I see you want that ball all to yourself. When you're finished, will you give it to Ken?" This kind of dialogue introduces both children to the idea of taking turns in a way that does not shame them. This won't always have a happy ending, but if you continually put your child's feelings into words for him, you'll be surprised how often he will rise to the occasion.

When the children seem especially calm and happy, you can use this time of peace to teach them how to take turns by playing simple games. Have each child take a turn:

- Hiding and finding a ball under a blanket.

- Rolling a ball back and forth (to illustrate the notion that what you share eventually comes back).

- Putting blocks into a pail and dumping them out.

- Stacking three blocks.

Our kids don't need our help to learn how to play. But they do need our help to learn how to play with others. At this age, give your son lots of social opportunities to try, fail, and then try again.

IMAGINARY FRIENDS

When other kids aren't around to amuse your son, he may surprise you by inventing his own imaginary playmate. The first time I met such a "friend," I was really quite shocked. I had taken my two-year-old son and his two-year-old friend, Lauren, to the park to play on the swings. Lauren first sat in one swing and was happily enjoying the ride while Joey ran around in circles for a while. Then suddenly, Joey came running across the park at full speed and threw his body, stomach first, on the swing next to Lauren. She became hysterical! Through her sobbing gasps I was finally able to figure out that Joey had jumped on top of her "friend," who was on the swing first. Of course, Joey wouldn't get off of this "friend," so we all left the park in varying emotional states: Lauren very upset, Joey laughing, and me completely confused.

Research shows that as many as 65 percent of children have imaginary friends, and the creation of such friends is associated with positive characteristics. For example, in comparison with children who don't have imaginary companions, those who do are more sociable, less shy, have more real friends, are more creative, and participate in more family activities. Imaginary companions also seem to help children learn social skills and practice conversations. In fact, one researcher found that they are powerful predictors that children will play happily in nursery school and will be cooperative and friendly with peers and adults.

So, there you have it. If your son begins to talk to thin air, or even ask for a second sandwich for his invisible friend, don't get alarmed. Apparently, it's a good thing!

Acting Like a Boy

Your son won't be quite sure if he is a boy or a girl until he's about three years old, but he's already learning a lot about gender roles—what it means to be male or female in a particular society. Although gender roles in America have become more flexible over the last fifty years, a large chunk of society still expects boys to wear pants, get dirty, play tough, and not cry. Girls, on the other hand, are expected to wear dresses (at least sometimes), play with dolls, stay clean, and be kind and quiet. Before we continue, let's take a look at some of the underlying reasons for this.

The roles assigned to males and females help children understand their gender identity. As males learn that they are boys, they want to know, "What does that mean?" They look around for ways to fit in and be accepted. Child development experts have witnessed how little boys who prefer to play dress-up learn rather quickly to pretend they like football so they are not ridiculed and shunned by the other boys. This awareness that boys do things differently than girls is tied in to the healthy process of self-discovery.

Long before they even know they are male or female, toddlers gravitate toward stereotypically male or female toys. To me, the most astonishing thing about this is the speed with which children learn these stereotypical roles.

I made a conscious effort to raise my children in a gender-neutral environment where any role (tough, soft, dirty, or clean) was accepted. I filled our backyard with toys for exploring all facets of life on an equal basis. That's why I was so surprised when I looked out the window one Saturday morning and saw my two-year-old son pushing the toy lawn mower around the yard, while our neighbor's two-year-old daughter pushed the toy baby carriage. Where did they learn this stuff?

Apparently, kids pick up cues about the sexes early and very rapidly. To test how two-year-olds connect gender with particular activities, future roles, and personality traits, researchers tried an interesting experiment. Given the limited level of verbal skills, researchers taught the young children to point to pictures of "Lisa" or "Michael" to indicate their responses. They found that the children thought Lisa liked to play with dolls, clean house, cook dinner, talk a lot, and never hit, while Michael liked to play with cars, build things, fight, and be loud, naughty, and make girls cry. They thought Lisa would grow up to clean the house and be a nurse or teacher, while Michael would mow the grass and be the boss.

WHERE DO THEY GET THESE IDEAS?

Do boys act like "boys" because they're hardwired at birth that way or because they learn male behavior from the world they live in? Nobody really knows for sure because there are strong arguments on both sides.

Some scientists believe this early grasp of gender roles is inborn and caused by differences in the brain created by hormones in the womb. Males are exposed to higher levels of androgen, and females to higher levels of estrogen. Some of this gender study is based on interesting research done with opposite-sex twins who naturally share the androgen and estrogen hormones. In these cases, the male tends to have more feminine attributes (lower levels of activeness, loudness, confidence, intensity, and selfishness) than his male peers, and the female twin shows higher masculine attributes (better spatial and mathematical abilities and increased dominance and sensation-seeking behavior) than her female peers. Researchers believe these results are due to the fact that androgen and estrogen hormones transfer from one fetus to another. This finding supports those who believe that at least some male-female differences are the result of hormone exposure in the womb and not the result of social conditioning alone.

Yet no one doubts that even if male/female behavior traits are inborn, the world a child lives in still has a mighty strong influence. Maggie Butterfield, director of community education at Children's Health Education Center at Children's Hospital of Wisconsin, says there is no doubt that as parents we are the ultimate role models for our children, and the way that we act our part as males or females will be imitated by our children—for both good and bad. "If Mom does all the indoor work and Dad does all the outdoor work," says Butterfield, "then our children will associate male behavior with the harder grunt work and females with the indoor care-taking work. So you might see more young girls playing 'house' while boys play construction worker.

"Of course, children will cross over these lines in their play because today they have more adult models who give them more options to imitate. One mom recently told me that her little girl packed up her backpack and said that she was going to the office.

This mom worked outside the home and gave her daughter a non-traditional model to imitate."

Still, even high-level corporate moms and stay-at-home dads scratch their heads in wonder when they see their children play in stereotypical gender roles. The fact is, say many child development experts, that these moms and dads are probably not as neutral in their encouragement of crossing gender lines as they think. Children learn, not only by the types of toys they play with, but also through the reaction of others when they play with it. Buying a son a doll is not the same thing as smiling at him when he plays with it. Very often, children will receive more positive rewards for doing gender-typical things, and this encourages them to repeat those behaviors.

In one study reported in *Child Development* in 1991, researchers Fagot and Hagan found that one-year-old boys and girls did not seem to care what toys they played with. Their play included dolls, puppets, and soft toys as well as trucks, cars, and blocks. However, when parents began to react more favorably to gender-typical toys during the second year, the children became more stereotypical in their choices. The boys, for example, received more positive reactions than girls for playing with transportation and building toys. The parents showed more interest and enthusiasm when joining in to play with toys that were more gender-specific. They found that parents tolerated some cross-gender play, but their positive reactions to such play declined steadily from about eighteen months on and declined faster for boys than girls.

Another study found that dads were the ones who most often rewarded their children (especially sons) for choosing gender-appropriate toys. In one experiment, preschool boys were given "girl" toys to play with and the girls were given "boy" toys. The researchers monitored the parents' reactions when they entered the room. The mothers were generally positive to both feminine and masculine play, often sitting down and joining in regardless of the type of toy. But the fathers reacted very negatively when they found their sons playing with feminine toys; they responded with frowns and sarcastic comments, and some even picked up the boy and physically moved him away from the kitchen set!

But parents aren't the only ones who influence a child's view of gender roles. Children who are in daycare, for example, are likely to spend long hours in the care of a female. The role model here is the nurturing, caring female. After spending weeks and months in this environment, it's unlikely that a little boy will say he wants to be a nursery school teacher. Or that a little girl will think about being a banker.

Playmates, too, are bound to influence gender ideas. In fact, in her book *A Field Guide to Boys and Girls,* author Susan Gilbert says that where attitudes about gender are concerned, playmates seem more influential than parents. She mentions an interesting study to make the point in which researchers observed groups of toddlers and preschoolers. They found the boys punished other boys by ignoring or teasing them for playing housekeeping, drawing, or engaging in other quiet activities. But boys laughed, cheered, or joined in when the other boys played with trucks or acted rambunctious. The caregivers praised all the children for their quiet play, but this praise had far less impact on the boys than on the girls. Other researchers found that if a boy picked up a feminine toy, the other boys would make fun of him and in some cases, even hit him. But when a girl played with a masculine toy, the other girls

SCIENCE SAYS

Even babies seem to prefer their own sex. Studies show that at the early age of six months, boys show increased attention to male faces, and in other studies researchers found that infants preferred to watch the pattern of biological motion produced by a same-sex child. The patterns were produced by attaching lights to the joints of a boy and a girl and filming the children walking in the dark. Slightly different patterns were produced because girls' wider hips give them a more rolling gait. The girls spent more time watching the movement of the female figures, and the boys watched the male figures.

usually ignored her (not as directly critical, but still not the response kids want from their playmates.)

In her work as the director of coummunity education at Children's Health Education Center at Children's Hospital of Wisconsin, Maggie Butterfield has seen the many ways that children learn gender roles. "As parents," says Butterfield, "we can't assume that we are the only adults affecting our children's idea of gender. The child's grandparents, siblings, aunts, uncles, childcare workers, baby-sitters, and playmates, all play a role. This is especially true in families where both parents work long hours outside the home." No matter how careful you are to encourage your son's sensitive side, you can be sure that everyone your child spends significant time with will also have an influence—and often that influence may encourage age-old stereotypes.

WHAT DO THEY LEARN?

The way that parents, caregivers, and playmates react to boys teaches them lots of things about how to be male. One of those things is how to be more independent than girls. Over and over, child development experts have watched parents comfort their daughters who are fearful or sad by holding them close and soothing them, while their sons are given a quick hug and an encouraging push to "get back out there." It is the boys who are expected and encouraged to play independently, to solve their own problems, and fight their own battles.

And apparently they get the message. Researchers studying children's behavior found that when mothers placed their thirteen-month-old babies in an unfamiliar room filled with toys to play with, the girls spent more time near their mother, came back to her more frequently, and maintained contact more continuously through touching, glancing, and talking. Boys were more likely to go farther from their mother, perhaps even to the farthest side of the room, to spend less time close to her, and to check in with her less frequently.

So why do parents encourage independence in their boys? I have to wonder if we're biologically programmed to do this given that even rhesus monkey mothers tend to reject their sons earlier than their daughters and force the young males to establish their own independence!

Whether by social habit or inborn instinct, I can see that there are advantages to raising an independent child, but from my point of view as a parent, there is also a drawback: independent boys are more difficult to discipline. People in the know say there's no doubt that boys are more likely to get into trouble and less likely to obey when they are told to stop doing something. One possible reason is their need for attention. Because they are generally left to play independently, they must devise ways to get their parents' attention. One sure way to bring a parent running is to play with the knobs on the stereo system, throw toys in the toilet, or draw on the walls with lipstick. When little boys do these things, they are considered "a typical boy."

THE MEANING OF GENDER

Here are a few easy tips for giving our kids a broad, accepting view of what it means to be male and female:

- Recognize the modeling you do. When it comes to gender development, the old adage is true: It's not what you say, it's what you do that counts. Let your son see you sharing household tasks such as washing dishes, mowing the lawn, making repairs, and shopping for food so he does not assume that some jobs are done only by men and others only by women.

- Expose your son to adults in nontraditional occupations. Let him see a male nursery school teacher and a female doctor.

- Monitor TV shows. When you see a show that uses gender stereotypes, either turn it off or play a game of retelling the story, placing the characters in different roles.

- Point out the biology of the sexes. While bathing your son, name his penis and tell him that only boys have a penis, girls do not. (Your son would not be the first to then ask everyone he sees if he or she has a penis and if he could see it!)

WHAT'S A PARENT TO DO?

After reading all this information about how toddlers learn how to be a boy or a girl, my bottom-line question is: Is it a bad thing when one- and two-year-olds learn stereotypical gender roles? It seems that the answer is a definite yes and no. "It's a bad thing," says Butterfield, "only when we try to determine that there is only one role our children can play. Our job is to expose our children to a variety of things that they have the capacity to do and to be successful at. Some of these are traditional roles, and some are not."

To do this for our children, we have to make a conscious effort and be aware that everything we do is being carefully watched and analyzed. (Not too much pressure!)

Learning how to be a boy takes time. It is a subtle back-and-forth dance between inborn tendencies and learned beliefs. It is remarkable to me that the gender beliefs picked up in these very early years can last a lifetime. So while it might be cute to hear a two-year-old say that only mommies can wash clothes, think how that same sentiment will sound to your boy's future wife!

Becoming a Little Man

As your son moves closer to his second birthday, you'll see that he's left babyhood behind in his dust. It's now full speed ahead to the preschool years and beyond, along with all the excitement and adventures you will share together as your little boy ultimately begins growing into a man.

MY BABY BOY

"I notice that my son and daughter definitely choose gender-specific toys. Travis always loves cars, trucks, rescue heroes, and Mackenzie naturally goes for the dolls and anything that can go on her arm like a bracelet. She also loves to play dress-up; she puts her dad's underwear around her neck and body and prances around the house. Travis is never interested in dress-up and never thinks of putting on my clothes, or my husband's, for that matter. But they are both equally cuddly to both me and their dad."

—Denise DePrima
Mother of 2-year-old Mackenzie and 5-year-old Travis

Epilogue

By now you should have a good sense of what adventures await you and your young son, along with advice and guidance on how to make the most of these early years—always keeping in mind the many factors that make little boys different from little girls.

Learning about these differences has helped me to better understand my own sons, and I hope the information will be useful to you as well. I now know why it was foolish to wish my high-wire son could be more like his calm and less aggressive sister. He is what he is, in large part because he is male. Realizing this makes his active personality (to put it nicely) less frustrating for me.

Of course, for every generalization, there are exceptions, and nothing stated in this book is absolute for all children. But knowing what "many" and "most" boys are like based on their body chemistry and the way their brains are wired gives us insights that I believe will help us all to be better parents.

In closing, I'd like to tell you how my own two sons have grown into manhood. Through the many stories about Matt and Joey that I've shared with you throughout the book (far more than they probably think is a good idea!) I'm sure you've noticed that they are each quite unique. Although I talk a lot about "boys" as a collective and similar group, obviously there are wide differences between each individual male child, and my two certainly make that point. Matt was my self-controlled and very cerebral son, while Joe was the far more impulsive one who tore through every day with abandon. Today, Matt is a nuclear engineer and an officer in the United States Navy. Joe attends college on a baseball scholarship and continues to amaze me with his boundless energy and athleticism. Their experiences growing up have given me a life full of wonderful memories that I have been happy to share with you.

As you raise your son, keep in mind that boyhood is a temporary state that goes by very quickly. It won't be long before you look back and wonder how that little blur of energy zipping by you so quickly turned into such a handsome young man.

Acknowledgments

The author would like to thank the following for their help in the preparation of this book:

Armin Brott, author of *The New Father: A Dad's Guide to the Toddler Years*.

Maggie Butterfield, director of community education at Children's Health Education Center/Children's Hospital of Wauwatosa, Wisconsin.

Freddie Curtis, director of Fashion Design and Fashion Merchandising programs, Harcum College in Bryn Mawr, Pennsylvania.

Cleveland Kent Evans, American Name Society.

Alice Sterling Honig, Ph.D., professor emerita of child and family studies in the College of Human Services and Health Professions at Syracuse University and a fellow of the American Psychological Association and the Society for Research in Child Development.

Susan Isaacs Kohl, preschool director, Lafayette, California, and author of *The Best Things Parents Do*.

Claire Lerner, LCSW, development specialist, Zero to Three, national nonprofit organization.

Stephen E. Muething, M.D., section director of clinical services at Cincinnati Children's Hospital Medical Center.

Maureen O'Brien, Ph.D., director of parenting and child development at The First Years, Inc., in Avon, Massachusetts.

Laurie Smith, interior designer, host of *Trading Spaces*.

My thanks also to Carole Beal of the University of Massachusetts Amherst, whose writing on gender development first sparked my interest in this fascinating subject. And to the authors of two books that were invaluable in my search for answers: Susan Gilbert, *A Field Guide to Boys and Girls*, and Michael Gurian, *Boys and Girls Learn Differently!*

I would like to acknowledge Kirk Kazanjian of Literary Productions. Right from the start, he has been the brains and the energy behind this project.

And a special thanks to Marilyn Galluccio, director of Enchanted Garden Nursery School in Hawthorne, New Jersey, and to all the moms and dads who shared their thoughts about raising little boys and girls: Lisa Cannizzo, Denise DePrima, Luisa DeSavino, Elizabeth Elia, Shawn Elton, Nancy Finch, Grace Foy, Kristen Garza, Jim Hauser, Kim Hauser, Kim Marone, Tina Marie and Dominick Martone, Shelley Sasaki, Ken Schultz, Cassandra Tiensivu, Melda Yildiz, and Tamalyn Roberts.

Appendix A

Editor's note: To download growth charts, please do the following:

CHART #1
1. Go to www.cdc.gov/growthcharts
2. Select "Clinical Growth Charts"
3. Locate "Set 2: Clinical charts with 3rd and 97th percentiles"
4. Under "Birth to 36 months (3rd–97th percentile)" click on
   view/download PDF for Boys Length-for-age and Weight-for-age
   (Black and White) 41KB

CHART #2
1. On same page, scroll down to "Children 2 to 20 years (3rd–97th
   percentile)
2. Locate "Boys Stature-for-age and Weight-for age" and click on
   view/download PDF (Black and White) 79KB

Birth to 36 months: Boys
Length-for-age and Weight-for-age percentiles

NAME _____

RECORD # _____

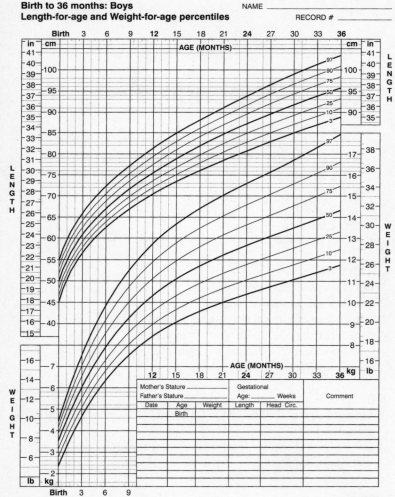

Published May 30, 2000 (modified 4/20/01).
SOURCE: Developed by the National Center for Health Statistics in collaboration with
the National Center for Chronic Disease Prevention and Health Promotion (2000).
http://www.cdc.gov/growthcharts

SAFER · HEALTHIER · PEOPLE™

2 to 20 years: Boys
Stature-for-age and Weight-for-age percentiles

NAME _____

RECORD # _____

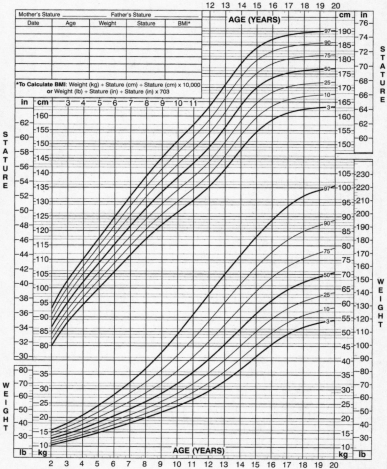

*To Calculate BMI: Weight (kg) ÷ Stature (cm) ÷ Stature (cm) x 10,000
or Weight (lb) ÷ Stature (in) ÷ Stature (in) x 703

Date	Age	Weight	Stature	BMI*

Published May 30, 2000 (modified 11/21/00).
SOURCE: Developed by the National Center for Health Statistics in collaboration with
the National Center for Chronic Disease Prevention and Health Promotion (2000).
http://www.cdc.gov/growthcharts

SAFER · HEALTHIER · PEOPLE™

Sources

Chapter 1

Carole Beale, *Boys and Girls, The Development of Gender Roles*. New York: McGraw-Hill, 1994.

Elise Yong, "Oh, Baby, Give Me a Boy," *Record News*, September 24, 2003, A12.

Chapter 2

Howard Moss, "Early Sex Differences and Mother-Infant Interaction," *Sex Differences in Behavior*. Eds. R. C. Friedman, R. M. Richart, and R. L. van De Wiele. New York: John Wiley & Sons, 1974. p. 149–63.

Edward Tronick and Lauren Adamson, *Babies as People*. New York: Macmillan, 1980.

Chapter 3

Magnus Domellof, Bo Lonnerdal, Kathryn G. Dewey, Roberta J. Cohen, L. Landa Rivera, Olle Hernell, "Sex Differences in Iron Status During Infancy," *Pediatrics* 110 (2002), p. 545–552.

Edward Tonick and John Cohn, "Infant-Mother Face-to-Face Interaction, Age and Gender Differences in Coordination and the Occurrence of Miscoordination," *Child Development* 60 (1989), p. 85–92.

Chapter 4

P. A. Katz and S. Boswell, "Sex Role Development and the One-Child Family," *The Single-Child Family*. Ed. T. Falbo. New York: Guilford Press, 1984. p. 63–116.

Lindsey Tanner, "TV May 'Rewire' Brains of Very Young Children," *The Record*, April 5, 2004, A7.

D. Tuller, "Poll Finds Even Babies Don't Get Enough Rest," *The New York Times*, March 30, 2004, F5.

Chapter 5

Carole Beale, *Boys and Girls, The Development of Gender Roles*.

T. Bower, *Development in Infancy* 2nd ed. San Francisco, CA: Freeman, 1982.

J. Condry and S. Condry, "Sex Differences, A Study of the Eye of the Beholder," *Child Development* 47 (1976), p. 1417–25.

L. Ellis and L. Ebertz, *Males, Females, and Behavior*. Westport, CT: Praeger, 1998.

B. Fagot and R. Hagan, "Observation of Parent Reactions to Sex-Stereotyped Behaviors, Age, and Sex Effects," *Child Development* 62 (1991), p. 617–628.

Susan Gilbert, *A Field Guide to Boys and Girls*. New York: HarperCollins, 2000.

Susan Goldberg and Michael Lewis, "Play Behavior in the One-Year-Old Infant, Early Sex Differences," *Child Development* 40 (1969), p. 21–31.

Melissa Healy, "Germ Warfare," *Record News*, April 6, 2004, F1.

E. Hetherington, M. Stanley-Hagen, and E. Anderson, "Marital Transitions," *American Psychologist* 44 (1989), p. 303–12.

D. Kimura, *Sex and Cognition*. Cambridge, MA: MIT Press, 1999.

D. Kuhn, S. Nahs, and L. Brucken, "Sex Role Concepts of Two- and Three-Year-Olds," *Child Development* 49 (1978), p. 445–51.

Charles Schaefer and Theresa DiGeronimo, *Toilet Training Without Tears*. New York: Signet, 1997.

M. Siegal, "Are Sons and Daughters Treated More Differently by Fathers Than by Mothers?" *Developmental Review* 7 (1987), 183–209.

Index